BEYOND
THE
BREATH

EXTRAORDINARY MINDFULNESS
THROUGH WHOLE-BODY
VIPASSANA MEDITATION

BEYOND
THE
BREATH

EXTRAORDINARY MINDFULNESS
THROUGH WHOLE-BODY
VIPASSANA MEDITATION

by
Marshall Glickman

JOURNEY
EDITIONS

Boston • Rutland, Vermont • Tokyo

First published in 2002 by Journey Editions, an imprint of Periplus Editions (HK) Ltd., with editorial offices at 153 Milk Street, Boston, Massachusetts 02109.

Library of Congress Cataloging-in-Publication Data

Glickman, Marshall
  Beyond the breath : extraordinary mindfulness through whole-body Vipassana meditation / Marshall Glickman.-- 1st ed.
     p. cm.
  Includes index.
  ISBN 1-58290-043-4 (pbk.)
    1. Vipaâyanâ (Buddhism) 2. Meditation--Buddhism. 3. Religious life--Buddhism. 4. Buddhism--Doctrines. I. Title.

BQ5630.V5 G54 2002
294.3'4435--dc21

Distributed by

**North America, Latin America,
and Europe**
Tuttle Publishing
Distribution Center
Airport Industrial Park
364 North Clarendon, VT 05759-9436
Tel: (802) 773-8930
Tel: (800) 526-2778
Fax: (802) 773-6993

Asia Pacific
Berkeley Books Pte. Ltd.
130 Joo Seng Road
#06-01/03 Olivine Building
Singapore 368357
Tel: (65) 6280-1330
Fax: (65) 6280-6290

Japan & Korea
Tuttle Publishing
Yaekari Bldg., 3F
5-4-12 Ōsaki, Shinagawa-ku
Tokyo 141 0032
Tel: (03) 5437-0171
Fax: (03) 5437-0755

First edition
05 04 03 02 01 00   9 8 7 6 5 4 3 2 1

Design by Linda Carey
Printed in the United States of America

CONTENTS

DEDICATION

This book is dedicated to my mom, Anne Glickman. In honor

of her love, intellect, honesty, and indefatigable spirit.

She died of cancer at the age of 64, while I was working on this book.

She gave so much; my debt to her is incalculable.

PREFACE

WHY I WROTE THIS BOOK

L ike many so-called spiritual seekers, I started meditating when I was struggling and open to change. It was
my senior year in college and I was confused about what
to do after graduating. At the time, it seemed I had one of two
choices: either to follow my freedom-loving and searching side,
the one that studied philosophy, traveled during the summers,
and experimented with recreational drugs; or to heed my
success-is-real-important suburban New York Jewish upbring-
ing—the part of me that gunned for A's, knew my G.P.A. down
to the second decimal point, and could rattle off a list of the
country's top law schools. Ultimately, I abandoned my child-
hood plans to become a lawyer or a professional of any kind,
but it left me anxious. Looking for some peace of mind, I turned
to Zen meditation.

Zen promised a take-life-as-it-comes fluidity that I lacked
and a way to live well no matter what I did for a job. I was drawn
to Zen's quiet dignity, and my twenty-year-old self found its
mysterious methods appealing. I began meditating twenty to
thirty minutes a day alone in my dorm room.

Meditating was a real struggle at first. Simply staying still
for ten minutes was challenge enough—and then my ankles and
thighs would burn from sitting in the half-lotus position. By the
end of most meditation sessions, I was shaking, drenched in
sweat, and ready to pounce on the alarm clock. But I was
intrigued—and desperate—enough to stick with it. I liked the
heightened intensity meditation brought to moments I would

have otherwise thought of as uneventful. And I savored those times I could completely focus on one thing. Within a few months I was waking at 4:30 a.m. to sit with a local Zen group. In the evenings, I usually put in another hour by myself, doing two to three hours a day.

Meditating increased my concentration and clarity of thought. It made it easier to appreciate life's "simple" pleasures. After returning from early morning sittings, I'd watch the sun rise over Lake Michigan and be moved to tears or shouting by the beauty of the pastel display reflected off the water or jagged ice. Other times, seeing steam dance in a ray of sunlight could take my breath away.

At the time, I thought meditating was getting rid of my anxiety. In retrospect, I see that while it did quiet my mind some, I hadn't genuinely come to terms with what bothered me. Back then, I saw emotions (at least the negative ones) as something largely to be conquered. I eagerly lapped up books filled with stories of meditators having powerful, transforming experiences after years of cross-legged concentration or during intense retreats. Some accounts spoke of complete freedom from unhappiness. I became convinced my petty self could be transcended if I worked hard enough. So I buckled down, bent on—I'm embarrassed to say—the quick, it-could-happen-any-day-now enlightenment plan.

For seven years, Zen was my anchor. Meditating helped maintain my sanity while I worked a sixty-hour a week job, and it was my steady companion through a series of mostly unsuccessful or nonexistent relationships. I might forget to call a girlfriend, but I rarely missed a day of sitting. And while I might be reluctant to take a vacation, I regularly attended Zen retreats called *sesshins* (week-long, silent meditating-fests) which entailed sitting eleven to twelve hours a day.

During one sesshin, however, my Zen mooring was literally beaten loose by a Japanese Zen master and his wooden stick.

At this retreat, during a private meeting with the teacher, I complained of being unmotivated. ("Maybe," I said, "it's because I'm not in as much pain as I used to be.") In a flash, the teacher pulled me forward and smashed his *kyosaku* stick on my back. He stung me again and again with sharp blows as he told me to shout my koan. I hollered *REALLY LOUD* and long and lost track of the whacks, occasionally wondering why I didn't run or grab his stick.

Afterwards, I found my back badly bruised; between my shoulder blades sat a shiny purple-and-blue lump the size of a baseball. Oddly, it didn't hurt much, but I was dazed. The kyosaku is part of the Zen tradition, but I'd never heard about anything like this. Usually, one gets a few strategic swats on the back for a burst of energy. And in western countries, a meditator only gets hit if he requests it. This pummeling clearly went well beyond that and it sent me into a tizzy. I felt stuck between quitting the retreat and rejecting Zen or trying to understand what had happened. Unable to do either, I threw myself into meditating and tried blocking out everything else.

Maybe the teacher had intuited that I was ripe for such a pounding; maybe in Japan he had received many such floggings from his teacher and he didn't realize he was overstepping cultural boundaries. I can still wrestle with the ethics of that whomping. Was it wrong? On principle, I know it was. But as it turns out, he did me a favor.

During that retreat, even as I continued to flounder, my concentration became very strong as I clung to my koan. Eventually the combination of struggle and effort wore me down and I just gave up and went limp. Then, everything dropped away except for an awareness of pure, formless, universal energy—what some, I think, would call God. It's hard to say how long this "view" lasted, but I felt no doubt about its reality. It wasn't a thought; it was something I had come upon. My overwhelming reaction was of awe and then, later, a big "aha." Now I knew what the expression "the cosmic dance" really meant. Infinite, all-pervasive energy underlies everything and is everything. We may think we do our own thing, we may even exercise our "own" will, but I saw that our life and all things are fleeting, ever-changing expressions of this energy.

I got no sense of whether this energy was benevolent. As far as I could tell, it simply was/is (if in a dizzyingly awesome way). But its very existence had implications. It confirmed that making spiritual matters central in my life was my best—and only real—choice. It gave me a more powerful conviction than ever that an Ivy League career didn't matter, but that working on myself and helping others did.

Despite the gain for my pain and gratitude for the expansive view, I didn't conclude that the smashed-back route was the way to go. I recognized how unbalanced I was. My lump helped me see that I had turned enlightenment into a goal as though it were an achievement that could be won. One of the reasons I had started meditating in the first place was to learn to be more process- and less accomplishment-oriented. Yet, clearly I hadn't changed; I was as results-oriented as ever.

I didn't disavow Zen or stop meditating, but I did soften up a bit. I became more open-minded about other spiritual paths (and nonpaths). I faced the fact that despite years of serious meditating, I was still often inflexible, defensive, and hard-edged. Simply being able to comfortably recognize those flaws was a change itself; I doubt it was a coincidence that around that time I found myself in a healthy relationship, eventually marrying and having children.

Echoing the generally gentler me, I started doing yoga and changed how I meditated. Instead of working on a Zen koan, I'd just sit as still as possible, trying to be aware of whatever presented itself. I drifted toward a popular form of Thai-inspired vipassana meditation, taught at the Insight Meditation Center.

Vipassana takes a softer approach than Zen (at least as Zen is usually practiced). There are no prodding sticks, loving-kindness meditations are part of the practice, problems in the community are openly addressed, and an egalitarian spirit runs through the organization. Instead of a single head teacher, different teachers take turns leading retreats. And unlike Zen, which seems to attract more men, vipassana retreats draw a balanced gender mix.

Though the gentleness and community's openness was welcome, I found that the form of Insight meditation I first practiced didn't take me as deep into the mind-body complex as the type of vipassana meditation I advocate in this book. It also didn't foster the keen awareness of emotions, which seems crucial for greater sensitivity and self-understanding. While all forms of vipassana meditation aim to bring its practitioners to complete mindfulness, in my experience one method does a better job of this than others (detailed in chapters 4 and 9).

At some point, it became clear (with some prodding from those close to me) that I needed to do more than just meditate. Although most acquaintances probably saw me as a peaceable, friendly, environmental activist, my aggressive and insensitive side indicated unexplored and unreconciled territory. I began psychotherapy with a woman whose even-handed and sympathetic directness helped show me how I ran from uncomfortable feelings. Although this therapist has no ostensible spiritual leanings or training, in many ways her advice echoed Eastern teachings: the best way to learn about my feelings, she advised, was simply to feel them.

Some months after beginning therapy, I accidentally learned about a different, lesser-known (at least in this country) form of vipassana which is often identified with its main teacher, S.N. Goenka. While Mr. Goenka refers to the method he teaches simply as "vipassana," it could be called sensation-based or whole-body vipassana, as the practice directs meditators to focus on sensations throughout their body. I didn't know this, though, before signing up for my first Goenka-style course. And once I discovered his method was different from what I expected, I was initially annoyed. For the first few days, I ignored his instructions, preferring what I thought of as meditating without any method or agenda. Yet, soon after giving the sensation-based technique a try, I recognized Mr. Goenka was really on to something.

It quickly became clear that sensation-based vipassana fostered better moment-to-moment awareness. It gave a way of experiencing emotions directly and nonverbally so they weren't overwhelming or alienating. Accessing the mind via the body made it easier to work with psychological scars that surfaced; it narrowed the gap between what is normally considered conscious and unconscious. And without any deliberate effort, my heart opened wider than it ever had. I've always tended to be more head- than heart-oriented, so discovering a spontaneous compassion told me I'd truly found something. I left the course excited and impressed by the technique, which continued to have an effect well beyond the normal, few-weeks-after-retreat glow.

Subsequent vipassana retreats deepened and expanded upon my initial experiences. They've brought greater insight into the unsubstantial, fleeting nature of life, a deeper, wordless recognition that we indeed own nothing, an understanding of how we multiply or can reduce negative states of mind, and an enlarged sense of internal spaciousness—leaving enough room for experiencing even anxious, angry, or fearful feelings without them taking the joint over. These realizations came gently, more like a dawning than a lightning bolt.

Incorporating sensation-based vipassana into my daily life has changed my inner world; it's lessened and turned down the volume on repetitive, unhelpful thought patterns, put me more at ease, and helped me become a more caring person. I'm not implying I'm beyond neurotic wheel-spinning, cantankerous behavior, or falling into old habits, but even while I'm in the midst of those difficulties, there's often still a measure of freedom I didn't have before. And when I do get overwhelmed or irritable, I'm better able to catch myself and am more apt to quickly apologize if I've hurt someone. Giving attention to my actual feelings has added a depth, calm, and clarity to lessons learned in psychotherapy (enough so, that I eventually, comfortably stopped therapy).

Yet, obviously, I'm no spiritual master. So you may be wondering, am I qualified to teach this method? Well, no . . . but then again, I don't see myself as a teacher. I believe there's a big difference between writing about wisdom and instructing others in person. A teacher should be, if not the perfect embodiment of his or her teachings, at least significantly closer to living it than the rest of us; a writer only needs to be near perfect on the page and direct you to an excellent teacher.

Alas, I fall short as the perfect writer too, but at least I'm qualified for this job. Partly because I've been writing for many years, and partly, ironically, because of my very lack of spiritual aptitude. As a seasoned journeyman who's tried different methods, read many of the best known books on Buddhism, and absorbed an American-influenced Buddhism from the trenches, I have insight into the ways many of us tend to misunderstand the Buddha's teachings.

It's been said that we learn more from our mistakes than our successes—and I think that's true—but only if we eventually have success; otherwise we just keep making the same mistakes over and over. If I hadn't been around the spiritual block before coming across this variety of vipassana, I wouldn't know just how lucid and exceptional Mr. Goenka's method is. And I wouldn't have become so devoted to finding out why it works so well (the answer to that takes up much of this book) or been so careful to clearly explain Buddhist principles so everyone can easily understand them.

In the few years I've been practicing sensation-based vipassana, I've made more progress and formed a much deeper understanding of Buddhism than in the previous sixteen years of doing other types of meditation. While I may have been unusually dense, this only highlights how effective this method is.

I used to be cynical about the very idea of happiness, convinced it could only apply to someone who lacked depth. Now I see I was totally wrong. The Buddha taught a sophisticated yet direct way to complete, unshakeable contentment. While I've got a long ways to go before mastering the complete or unshakeable part, I've never been happier. And I feel so grateful for that grace, I want to share it.

After I first recognized the effectiveness and ingenious simplicity of this mediation technique I found myself thinking, "This is awesome! Brilliant! This must be how the Buddha meditated!" Sometimes these thoughts were followed by, "How come I'd never heard about this before?"

This book exists so that fewer people will say just that.

AN ANCIENT PRACTICE FOR RIGHT NOW

The religion of the future will be a cosmic religion. It should transcend a personal god and avoid dogma and theology. Buddhism answers this description. If there is any religion that would cope with modern scientific needs, it would be Buddhism.
  —*Albert Einstein*

I t's tempting to get on a soapbox and proclaim why Buddhism is so needed at this troubled moment in history. The Buddha's path offers a time-tested, simple, yet powerful way to peacefulness, unconnected to dogma or celestial promises. It seems the perfect antidote for the frayed nerves, rampant materialism, and epidemic cynicism that are now so prevalent. Yet, while nearly everyone is disturbed by the state of the world, while nearly everyone bemoans a society that pushes what really matters—love, morality, and wisdom—to its margins, to hear someone gripe about it is tiresome; it quickly sounds like nagging.

Personal troubles, however, are a different story. Whether it's our friend's, a celebrity's, or even a stranger's problem, we can hardly get enough. And of course when it comes to our own problems, we're totally captivated—even while they drive us crazy. "How can I get rid of these beasts?" we wonder. "What can be done about this gnawing in my belly?"

These were the questions the Buddha asked himself. What caused his uneasiness and confusion? To find the answers, he worked like a scientist, making no presumptions and observing the truth within himself as objectively as possible. Eventually, he found what he was looking for: total freedom and inner peace, a resolution to the human dilemma. As some marketing whiz might put it, he took stress reduction to its omega point. Then, with an open hand, he offered his remedy to anyone who was interested. He knew whoever followed it could find the contentment he did—and if done en masse, would give us that harmonious society we all long for (without the sermons).

A BRIEF HISTORY

As a renowned historical figure, the Buddha is naturally surrounded by legends and competing beliefs. There are some basic facts, though, that most everyone agrees upon: so we might as well start there. First, he was a man, not a divine being, born Siddhartha Gautama in northern India. His father was either a king, a prince, or a clan chief. In any case, his dad had power and wealth and made sure his only son had it good: fine food and clothes, dancing courtesans, athletic training, and the best education. Yet, despite these advantages, Siddhartha found he wasn't really content. Seeking to find out why, he gave up his privilege and possessions and set out on a spiritual search. He studied with wise men and ascetics, fasting, prostrating, cogitating, and meditating. Though he mastered each technique and pushed himself mercilessly, he didn't find the peace he sought—until he set out on his own. Then, while meditating under the now-famous Bodhi tree, he found complete enlightenment, unbounded wisdom, total contentment, and lasting happiness. It was as though he roused from a deep sleep and was awake for the first time.

After absorbing this new vista for a while, the Buddha began teaching others what he had learned, so they too could find peacefulness. He laid out a prescription, best known as the Noble Eight-fold Path. When asked to sum up his teachings in the simplest terms possible, he said: "Abstain from unwholesome deeds, perform wholesome ones, and purify your mind."

After this, things get a bit messy, especially for those interested in reproducing the Buddha's results for themselves. The Buddha's fundamental insights—that life is suffering, that nothing is permanent, that there is no self—are widely agreed upon by Buddhists of all stripes. So is the need to follow moral guidelines and meditate. But how exactly did the Buddha meditate?

It seems there will never be a definitive answer to this question—though the sensation-based method of vipassana that S.N. Goenka teaches has a legitimate claim on being that original method. Buddhism in Burma, where Mr. Goenka learned this method, has flourished for over a thousand years, largely untouched by the changes the practice underwent as it spread eastward into China, Tibet, and Japan. This original practice is grounded in the ancient Buddhist texts called the Pali Canon. This collected work is a record of what the Buddha did and taught during his lifetime, including how to meditate. Using these words and other references in the Canon, one can make a reasonable claim that the practice Mr. Goenka teaches is either the exact method the Buddha himself used or one he'd advocate for lay people (see chapter 9 for details).

Like most ancient texts, the Pali Canon is open to interpretation (or elaboration). And based on different interpretations, a variety of Buddhist sects and schools of meditation have formed. Ironically, even within Buddhism itself, as each of us sets out in the spiritual marketplace, we face the same situation the Buddha himself did. For when Siddhartha left his palace, he encountered a world of wandering yogis, rishis, and philosophers, all making claims to the truth. Having sampled a variety of these wares myself, trying different types of meditation, therapy, and yoga before finally discovering this extraordinary practice, I find I want to shout in that market square, "Hey check this one out, I've tried others and they're good, but wow, this is great!" For it's the effectiveness and transformative power of sensation-based vipassana (and not its pedigree) that makes me eager to share it.

Apparently, I'm not the only one who feels this way. It seems many alumni of S.N. Goenka's courses feel compelled to pass on the benefits. Almost solely through word of mouth this method has spread throughout the world. In 1969, when Mr. Goenka left his teacher, Sayagyi U Ba Khin, to give a 10-day course in India to his ill mother and a few acquaintances, no one outside of Burma practiced this method. Mr. Goenka was a successful businessman with no students; he knew fewer than 100 people in the mostly Hindu and Muslim country. Yet, somehow, people started flocking to him. Seekers of all religious stripes from all over India and the whole world asked him to lead courses. Before long, he had taught his method to thousands of people. Then tens of thousands.

Determined to bring this technique home, students of Mr. Goenka began opening retreat centers across the globe. At this writing, there are more than eighty meditation centers worldwide, serving 50,000 retreatants a year. In addition, an estimated 10,000 prisoners have taken 10-day courses while still behind bars. This prison program, which started in a large Indian jail in

1994, has proven very successful and spread to other penal institutions in India, Taiwan, and the U.S. Inmates who stick with the method report being more peaceful and show dramatically lower recidivism rates. As Lucia Meijer, who runs the prison program in the state of Washington, said, "The technique can be characterized as a mental detox."

To maintain the purity of this practice, Mr. Goenka's organization is funded in an unusual way. In the tradition of the Buddha, who freely passed on his teachings, all courses (including room and board) are offered without charge. Teachers receive no compensation and facilities are paid for only by donations. After finishing a retreat, most participants make a contribution in the spirit of allowing others to benefit from the method. Yet there is no pressure to give or suggested minimums. You contribute as you can and feel moved to. And donations are only accepted from people who have completed a course.

WHAT'S AHEAD

Before taking a course, obviously you need to be motivated to do so. So this book is largely devoted to explaining both why it makes sense to practice this method and why it works so well. One reason is easy to explain: Mr. Goenka makes it clear that a meditation practice shouldn't stand on its own, separate from the rest of the Buddha's advice. To really change, we need to make efforts beyond just the meditation cushion. This isn't late-breaking news, but it's a message that has often been lost or not made explicit.

The Buddha clearly recommended a whole-life and ethical commitment. If we follow only part of his plan, we can't expect to get the full results, just as you wouldn't expect to lose much weight or become healthier if you only jog or do calisthenics, but don't also give up junk food.

Another strength of Mr. Goenka's presentation of Buddhism is that it focuses on the essentials of the Buddha's path. S.N. Goenka is a family man and learned this method while he was an active businessman with many responsibilities. His teacher, Sayagyi U Ba Khin, also had a big family and enormous responsibilities as a high-level government official in Burma. At one point in his career, U Ba Khin held up to four cabinet positions while maintaining his duties as a meditation teacher. So while U Ba Khin and Goenka's teachings are faithful to the Buddha's, there's nothing extraneous in their advice, making it well suited for those who never plan to put on a robe or shave their head.

Still, several bigger questions remain, such as, why is the Buddha's prescription so healing in the first place, and why is this particular method of meditation so effective? Or why do we need to adopt a whole-life approach and act ethically in order to be happy? Answering these questions comprises the bulk of this book. And assuming I've done my job well, the explanations should make plain not only why the Buddha and this technique are really on to something, but also give us insights into how to apply the Buddha's wisdom to situations he never explicitly discussed.

To do this, I've relied heavily on scientific findings. While this may initially strike some as inappropriate, it's hard to imagine the Buddha minding. In many ways, Gautama was the consummate scientist: he discovered a natural order that we must be aligned with if we are to find peacefulness. Why shouldn't many scientific discoveries be applicable to what the Buddha learned, even if the scientific research was done without any spiritual implications in mind? Darwin's theory of evolution, for example, which has weakened so many religions, actually dovetails well with many of the Buddha's insights. For instance, an evolutionary-developed sense of right and wrong suggests the importance of heeding our moral instincts, without implying that these intuitions were handed to us from an absolute power or that we should be judgmental of others who don't recognize this themselves.

Comparative religion scholar Huston Smith has noted that historically one of the functions of religion has been to explain why the world works the way it does. Given how successful the scientific method has been at providing mechanistic explanations, it's not surprising that science has become, in many ways, the de facto religion of our time—inheriting some roles it's not well suited for. So the more clearly I can show the scientific validity of the Buddha's path and this meditation technique, the more confidence our twenty-first century minds are likely to have in it. By relying on science in this way, I'm not implying that the Buddha's truth requires scientific validation, for indeed his ultimate realization is beyond the scope of science. Only that science can be a valuable tool for understanding Buddhism better.

Approaching Buddhism through scientific principles can help secularize ideas that may initially sound exotic, off-putting, or out-dated. Karma, for example, is often misunderstood, yet making use of recent neurochemical findings, we can see how our karma can be understood as our unconscious. We also see that our unconscious is not a static thing—not *the* unconscious—which we must endure as a hunchback must make due with their lump, but a dynamic process that is accessible and changeable with the right awareness. Other neurochemical research and evolutionary insights help explain many traditionally puzzling Buddhist conundrums, such as (to name but a few) what Buddhists mean when they say there is no self, why you needn't be a vegetarian to be a Buddhist, and why we easily get confused by and addicted to pleasure. If a monk or religious leader pointed out that pleasure can be addicting without first explaining the biochemistry of it, we're likely to think he's an extremist.

In the pages that follow, I hope to show that "abstaining from unwholesome deeds, performing wholesome ones, and purifying your mind" isn't an old-fashioned philosophy, but an effective way to become truly content, regardless of your beliefs or religion. Presented in a whirlwind as I've done in the last few paragraphs, it might sound as though I'm simply replacing confusing Eastern ideas with complicated scientific ones, but when the science is not condensed, it's quite accessible.

There has been very little written for a popular audience about S.N. Goenka's approach to Buddhism and meditation. One exception is *The Art of Living*, written by an assistant teacher of Goenkaji, as Goenka's students often call him. *The Art of Living* is based on the discourses Mr. Goenka gives at a 10-day retreat—except without detailing how to actually do the type of meditation he teaches. Not surprisingly, *The Art of Living* does an excellent job presenting the essentials of the Buddha's path and is much beloved. Throughout the book Mr. Goenka emphasizes a nonsectarian approach, yet his teachings are still presented mostly within a historic Buddhist framework, often using ancient Buddhist terms and traditional parables. This is as it should be, particularly since Mr. Goenka is the leading guardian of an invaluable treasure that had almost been lost. But much can be gained from also considering this technique and essential teachings from an interdisciplinary, western perspective, as well as from explicitly explaining how to do the method.

Until now, the only way to learn this technique was to complete a 10-day, silent retreat at a vipassana center. That is still the best way to absorb and appreciate this method. In fact, the ultimate aim of this book is that those new to this type of meditation will try a course. Although I offer instructions, learning the technique on your own isn't truly a substitute for the retreat experience.

So why include instructions at all? For starters, it makes it much easier to explain why the technique works so well. With only vague how-to references, it's more difficult to clearly distinguish how sensation-based vipassana is different from other types of meditation and why it's so effective. The second reason to include instructions is that one can be gradually introduced to the method. Obviously not everyone will be ready to sign on for a 10-day course after reading these pages—especially since it's unlikely that there is a retreat center near you (there are only six main centers in North America, all located in rural areas). That means many who are exposed to this method will never end up trying it, never getting a visceral sense of how it works and feels. It's one thing to read about the method and it's quite another to actually experience it. Even though practicing on your own is unlikely to give you as intense or as vivid an experience or understanding as you'd get from a retreat, it's still a taste. My ardent hope is that this book can whet your appetite and help you become comfortable with sensation-based vipassana so you make it part of your life, begin to understand why it's so helpful, and then, if possible, take a course.

PART 1

BUDDHIST BASICS

Before learning how to meditate, it's important to have some background. What is the goal of Buddhism and what role does this method of meditation play in the Buddha's prescription for happiness?

The next three chapters are designed to give a sense of context. First, through a jargon-free explanation of the Buddha's basic approach. Then, by briefly highlighting how paying attention to sensations dovetails with that strategy. And, last, by pointing out how the various aspects of the Buddhist path support each other. Ideally, this should be helpful both for those new to Buddhism, as well as those who are experienced meditators, especially if you're familiar with another tradition.

CHAPTER 1

HOW CHANGE CHANGES EVERYTHING

---

*The experience of impermanence (anicca), when properly
developed, strikes at the root of one's physical and mental ills
and removes gradually whatever is bad in him. . . . This experience is not reserved for men who have renounced the world
for the homeless life.*

—*Sayagyi U Ba Khin*

I f the known universe came with a handbook, rule number
one would be "everything changes." All is in motion.
Nothing stands still.

The smallest subatomic particles known to physicists, the
so-called building blocks of our world, zip around at incompre-
hensible speeds, darting in and out of existence. Atoms and
molecules, which are made of these wee particles, vibrate,
dance, and reconfigure. Ditto for our cells, which constantly
break down and regenerate: our stomach lining replaces itself
every five days, our skin once a month, and our bones every
three months.

Children grow; grandparents die. The earth moves around the sun; the sun whips around the galaxy. And the universe is expanding—or perhaps contracting. No matter which direction you look—up or down, at the big or the small, to the old or the young—the universe is fluid. There is no real solidity anywhere.

Since everything changes, nothing can be permanent. Leave bread out for a week and it grows stale and moldy, prey to fungus, humidity, oxidation, and a variety of other chemical processes. Toss the loaf outside, and soon enough it will turn into soil. Similarly, neglect your house for a few years and it too will start to deteriorate; its paint will flake, the roof will sprout a leak, the sill will rot. Do nothing for a few decades and the building will crumble, eventually leaving no traces at all. This is obvious enough, almost too mundane to mention—until we pay closer attention. Then we see that change is the opposite of mundane. It's what makes every moment new and different. It's what makes the world as we usually experience it unsatisfying, giving us an impetus to learn a better way. And of course it provides us with the ultimate motivator and drama: death.

On his deathbed, the Buddha said, "Decay is inherent in all compounded things." Clearly he wanted us to know this is an important principle. He knew once we recognize that change is constant and inescapable and make that understanding part of our awareness, we will relax our grip on life and focus on what really matters.

How can an awareness of change do that? Essentially the same way an appreciation of death can. After someone close to us dies or when we squarely face our own demise, we get perspective and become softer. We remember that we don't get to keep anything; so why devote ourselves to collecting things? Why build up our ego or get worked up about mishaps when eventually everything slips through our fingers anyhow? Being present, appreciative, and kind seem the natural and obvious way to go.

Overwhelmed and distracted by our emotions and busyness, we usually forget this bigger perspective. Ironically, this happens in large part because we miss the details of our life; we aren't aware of what is actually happening moment to moment.

Normally, we have a fairly crude appreciation of what we're experiencing and feeling at any given time. If someone asks us how we're doing, we'll usually say "okay" or "fine." If they're an intimate friend and ask how we're *really* doing, we'll report something like we're nervous, psyched, sad, frustrated, or proud. These general dispatches are accurate enough in a summing-up way, but they only partially capture what's happening in the moment.

After meditating a lot, your awareness can become so sensitive that you're very attuned to the subtlety of each instant. When this happens, you witness how insubstantial and fleeting every moment is. We are forever in a radical state of becoming and dissolving. Each moment passing even as it is happening. Sharpen our awareness even further, to meditation master level, and we'd see (as cognitive research confirms) that consciousness is not continuous. What we normally call a moment is actually comprised of many much faster "mini" moments, each rapidly appearing and disappearing. This happens so quickly, though, that we experience a steady state of consciousness, just as a movie appears seamless even though it's made of many quickly flashed still photos.*

---

* According to the ancient Buddhist text, the Abhidhamma, it takes seventeen mind-moments for a cognitive experience to register. Without that minimum of "sustained" contact, the experience won't be noticed. Research by experimental psychologists essentially confirms that a great deal of unconscious processing, measured in milliseconds, goes into creating a conscious moment. So if a sound (or any sensory input) doesn't engage these processes with enough repetitions, it remains below our level of conscious awareness—even though we may be aware of it at some level. This probably explains why subliminal advertising can be so effective (and is illegal): As you may remember from Psych 101, if the word "Coke" is flashed on a movie screen for a microsecond, much of the audience will head to the concession counter, even though they had no idea they'd seen the word.

Of course when most of us look around, things look pretty stable. Sure, we notice some change, especially if we look outside (right now, for instance, an insect is flying by, branches are swaying in the wind, and clouds are moving across the sky), but observing that kind of change is not likely to undermine our sense of solidity. It seems like just a little change in a mostly steady world.

The quickest way around this illusion of solidity (and it must be an illusion, if a shared one, since atoms and molecules are forever buzzing around here, there, and everywhere) is to turn inward and bypass our sense of sight and, more important, our ideas and interpretations about what we see.

Actually, the seeming stability of our vision doesn't just come from the eyeball or retina itself, but from the way these interact with assumptions supplied by various parts of our brain. Or, as molecular biologist and physicist Jeremy Hayward explained in layman terms: "the final image the brain makes available to your awareness is tremendously mixed up with your emotions, what you want to see and what you don't want to see, your preconceived ideas about the world, and what you expect to see and so on. This mixing up of your ideas with the message coming from outside you begins at the very moment the light hits your eye."

We don't see a mosaic of green, yellow, brown, and gray, but trees and a forest. Or, as Buddhist writer Stephen Batchelor notes, we don't come upon a frightening array of colors and shapes, but a snake in the grass. All our senses are like this (we hear a dog barking in the distance, not a hollow echoing sound), but vision, which involves our most complex sensory apparatus, is more intertwined with the conceptual parts of our brain than other senses. To see something involves considerably more cognitive processing than to smell something, which is our most direct sense.

Usually we think lots of cognitive processing is good; it implies a higher, more sophisticated understanding. Often this is true, especially when we're trying to analyze and figure things out, but it's a barrier for directly experiencing the way things are. Ideas are interpretations of reality. They frame and distort what we see. So experiencing reality sans ideas allows us to more directly apprehend things just as they are.

By trying a small experiment we can get a sense of how ideas give a misleading sense of structure and stability.

Consider your arm. First, just look at it; then think about it: What is an arm? This isn't a trick question; any thought or definition you come up with is fine. Most of us will think of something like "a dexterous limb attached to the shoulder that helps us pluck grapes or flag a cab." There's nothing particularly complicated or mysterious about it. An arm is an arm; its essence seems fairly easy to capture. Contemplating it in this way we get the sense that an arm is solid and real, something concrete we could refer to and hold.

Now close your eyes and try to clear your mind. Try to just *feel* one of your arms. Sit comfortably with your back straight and just observe. Let your arm relax, either hanging free or resting on your lap. Then examine whatever sensations are happening there. If a single sensation, say a throbbing in your triceps, dominates, then move your attention around a bit to other parts of the arm. This time you're trying not to think about or visualize your arm in any way; you're just examining it as if you were experiencing it for the first time. Give this at least a minute or so, keeping your eyes closed.

Experiencing your arm was obviously quite different than thinking about it. Even if it was difficult to focus solely on sensations without some images popping up, you probably noticed that there was a lot more happening there than a simple definition could capture. Maybe your arm felt heavy, maybe it pulsated or swirled, or possibly it felt as though it were burning. Whatever you experienced, no doubt the sensations kept changing and didn't fit the image we normally have when we think "arm." This brief exercise suggests that our arm—and indeed our whole being—isn't the solid, stable entity we usually imagine it to be. It shows how what we call me or myself is a constantly changing phenomenon that doesn't stay still for a moment and doesn't have distinct boundaries. It also shows, or at least hints at, how sensations can give a direct, experiential knowledge of some basic truths the Buddha wanted us to see: transience, lack of self, and the futility of grasping after experiences.

Thinking tends to have the opposite effect. Thoughts seem to seize and harden the ephemeral and amorphous. This happens for a couple of reasons. First, we think largely in images ("I see," we say when we understand something). And as cognitive psychologist Steven Pinker wrote, "Images are thumpingly concrete"; they automatically convey a sense of solidity. Second, ideas and concepts, even abstract ones, define; an idea identifies some point(s) or truth(s) in order to cut through ambiguity. So thoughts are accompanied by a feeling of precision and certainty. Whatever we're thinking, by definition, gives the impression (at least at that time) that our thinking is true and accurate. (Even thoughts expressing an uncertain sentiment are essentially definitive statements of uncertainty.)

The combination of images and definition gives our thoughts a firm sense of validity and stability. This in turn gives the sense that what we're thinking about has a fixed reality or kind of essence. When we think of water, for example, we attribute a flowing quality to it that is inherent in its existence. But where is that essential fluidity when you freeze it or boil it away?

This isn't a question reserved for philosophy majors. Our thoughts of "waterness," "iceness," and "steamness" give an order and shape to the world that belies its fragile, temporary, complex, and fuzzy nature. Ideas are static, but life is fluid. The sense of certainty that accompanies an idea covers over the magic that comes from experiencing life as a fleeting and delicate process. And when we attribute an underlying essence, thingness, or "me-ness" to ourselves, it makes us more rigid and inflexible. It draws us into protecting, glorifying, and fortifying a self-image. Instead of experiencing our life as an unfolding process, we try to frame it and grab it, blocking its flow. To paraphrase Mark Epstein in *Thoughts Without a Thinker*, we try to make nouns out of verbs.

The freeze-frame aspect of thought is so embedded in the way we think that we tend to miss how it causes us to see our very life as though it were a thing. We also miss how that life-as-thing approach often trips us up. While this misunderstanding will be considered more fully in the pages ahead, we can get a quick sense of the problems it creates by noticing what happens when we play sports. Say, for example, you're playing tennis and hit a fabulous return of serve. If you dwell on how wonderful your shot was, inevitably the next ball will whiz right by you. Or, similarly, if you drill a few forehands into the net and get stuck on the idea that you stink, your game will really fall apart. This pattern of thinking doesn't stop once we step off the court.

We're accompanied by an internal play-by-play announcer who is forever proclaiming the way things supposedly are and should be in our game of life. This announcer believes it's being helpful, but it doesn't realize the commentaries are ruining the game. Not only is it covering over the real action, but it's setting us up for disappointment, since the game itself rarely matches what's supposed to be happening.

To undermine this pattern and be truly immersed in the sport of life, we need to pay close attention to what is happening in each moment. Simply firing the announcer or vowing better concentration won't work; we need to create a whole mental culture that supports full awareness. Like becoming a good tennis player, we need sophisticated training, practice, and skill.

The Buddha's sport was happiness. He dedicated himself to it like few others before or since. And once he mastered it, he offered his training methods to anyone who was interested in developing their own game. Obviously, just liking the sport won't improve our skills. We must follow his regime. Happiness is a participatory sport.

So where do we start? Essentially with unhappiness; the Buddha tells us that if we want to get in shape, first we have to look in the mirror. Until we realize that some of the fabulous shots we thought we were hitting are actually landing out of bounds, we won't have much incentive to try a new coach.

CHAPTER 2

THE REAL STARTING POINT

Suffering is a big word in Buddhist thought. It is a key term and should be thoroughly understood.
—*Venerable Henepola Gunaratana,*
Mindfulness in Plain English

Discontentment, unhappiness, uneasiness. It doesn't matter what you call it, what disguise you put on it or what light you cast it in, discomfort, tension, and pain are the starting point for spiritual seekers of all stripes. It is where the Buddha himself began; first, as Siddhartha Gautama, who felt a restlessness so profound it drove him from his home and family. And later, after he found the ultimate peace he sought, it was where he began as a teacher: the opening words to the Buddha's first discourse, his first message to the world after his enlightenment speaks to this basic fact of life. This sentiment—which has become the single statement most associated with Buddhism and is now known as the First Noble Truth—has traditionally been translated as "Life is suffering."

In recent years, Buddhist scholars and teachers have tried to undo the public relations mishap of these early, slightly unfortunate translations. They point out that Buddhism isn't pessimistic; it is realistic. Or, if anything, it's optimistic, since the Buddha showed a way to end unhappiness—permanently.

So if the Buddha didn't say, "Life is suffering," what exactly did he say? *Dukkha*, the Pali word the Buddha used, does loosely translate into "suffering," but that suffering is not restricted to extreme pain. Of course agonizing pain is sometimes part of life. But pain and discomfort come in a variety of shades—from violent atrocities and gut-wrenching illnesses to mild irritations and vague worries.

To encompass the fuller range and constancy of our struggles, the usual, modern translation for dukkha is "pervasive dissatisfaction" or "off the mark." So the First Noble Truth more accurately (if more awkwardly) states, "Life is consistently dissatisfying" or "Life is never perfect." These translations highlight our everyday, underlying dis-ease, though I suppose they give short shrift to the pain of full-blown tragedies (how fitting that there isn't a perfect description of life's imperfection). Reflecting the many ways we are dissatisfied, dukkha has also been translated as "chronically frustrating," "disappointing," "hard to bear," "difficult," "hollow," "anguish," "stressful," and, based on the word's Sanskrit roots, "a wheel out of kilter."

Of course "Life is chronically disappointing" or "Life is off kilter" doesn't make for great ad copy either, but at least it has a compelling ring of truth. Still, it sounds so dismal, so un-American and unempowering. After hearing even the more accurate and nuanced version of the First Noble Truth, people often object: "Wait a minute. What about love, joy, fun, and friendship?!"

Of course the good, the true, and the beautiful do exist—or relatively so. Obviously some moments seem way nicer than others. These moments of grace are nothing to sneeze at, and as one becomes more peaceful, kind, and generous, they happen more frequently and "spontaneously." This is a good indicator that you're moving in the right direction. But if we examine even these best of times more closely, we find that something is always still a bit off.

Think about a great dinner party. Your best friends are there. You're in a groove; they're in a groove. Conversation is lively, loose, and intimate. At some point, you look around the table and are filled with a glow—ain't life sweet? Yet, invariably that feeling is accompanied by at least a tinge of sadness or anxiety, knowing things won't always be this way. Also, on closer inspection, how accurate is that glow-filled summation? Wasn't there at least some worry, bluster, and frustration during much of the evening? Did I say the wrong thing? Or, if I said just the right thing, did I get the kudos I was hoping for? What about that great story you didn't get to tell? Or the boring one your spouse did? A certain tension is still there, always there. Things aren't *just* right.

Okay, maybe you're not a party person. So put yourself at home, alone, with no work to do. Imagine you have the freedom to settle in on the couch and just relax one winter weekend. No one else is home and the phone is unplugged. You're just going to rest comfortably, taking that breather you've often longed for.

Odds are, within minutes you'll wish you were just a wee bit cozier; maybe you want a blanket or a fire in the hearth Soon after the fire is going, up pops the urge for a cup of tea. Then some biscuits. And then how 'bout some Mozart quartets? Or gosh, wouldn't it be swell to pick up a good novel? After a few pages you start nodding off or after reading about a sick heroine, you worry about your persistent cough—maybe it's really something serious. And so it goes. Naturally we ignore most of these impulses, if for no other reason than it's annoying to get up every five minutes, but the urges and restlessness are there. In fact, careful self-observation reveals an even greater, relentless antsiness.

Standing back and considering our impulses cumulatively, it hits us that we're so busy trying to get comfortable, we never actually relax. We're like a cartoon character so intent on finding the perfect sleeping position, he's up all night flopping around.

If you haven't made that careful investigation, you may be convinced that at least some of the time you were free of worries or dissatisfaction—a few pages of pure reading enjoyment or one exchange during the party when you and a friend felt like two souls uniting. Even if that were true, if you were to consider these irritation-free times as a percentage of our whole weekend, month, or life, things still look pretty dismal. Assuming our goal is happiness, it should make us wonder how effective our usual approach to living is (if you could call our usual way an approach, since rarely has it been thought through).

And we've been looking at the best of times—a great party, a relaxing, undemanding break. How many uninterrupted weekends with no pressing agendas, unwelcome phone calls, or chores do we get? How many truly great parties have you been to lately, or ever? Many are plainly awkward and disappointing.

Unconsciously, we wish a staff of attentive, eager-to-please, unnoticeable, and unpaid servants or robots could take care of these various "problems"—they could get us the tea we want, add wood to the fire, find us the perfect book, discreetly silence our spouse or enemy when needed, put the spotlight on us when we're telling a whale of a tale ("Will everyone shut up; he's talking!"). It doesn't take a Ph.D. in Life to know how far-fetched that fantasy is, but when we look for our happiness from people or things outside ourselves, essentially this is the premise we're working under.

Not surprisingly, statistics on material progress and happiness indicate that won't work. Since 1950, even after discounting the effects of inflation, the world has consumed twice as many goods and services as all previous generations put together. Yet regular surveys by the National Opinion Research Center of the University of Chicago show a decrease in overall happiness. We now make 2.5 times as much money as we did in 1960, yet since then our rate of divorce has doubled, teen suicide is up threefold, violent crime has increased fourfold, our prisoner population expanded fivefold, and the incidence of depression is ten times what is was 100 years ago.

In his book *How Much Is Enough?*, Alan Durning cites an extensive worldwide study that concluded there was no correlation between material prosperity and happiness. "Any relationship that does exist between income and happiness," writes Durning, "is relative rather than absolute." That is, the middle class in Nigeria or the Philippines are as happy as the middle class in West Germany or the U.S.—despite having lots less stuff. Ditto for the poorest and wealthiest groups in each country. So any pleasure we do get from buying stuff seems to hinge on one-upmanship, hardly a source of real fulfillment.

Try a little test. At this very moment, are you truly content? Don't respond right away, but really check in with yourself. Get quiet and observe not only your thoughts but what's happening in your body. Is there uneasiness or resistance? Odds are extremely high that something is bothering you, or at least things aren't quite right. The "problem" could be any of a zillion things that need adjusting, from needing a drink or having a bum knee to an unresolved spat with your partner, or sadness over not having a partner.

Doing this test once won't convince you of much: you could just be having a bad moment. So check in with yourself in about five minutes (after you've gotten your drink, an ace bandage for your knee, had a talk with your pal, or made any other myriad adjustments that could remedy problems from the previous check-in). Same result? Try again in fifteen minutes.

Then fifty minutes, then five hours, five days, and five months. Do this as many times as you feel necessary until you're convinced an undercurrent of discontent is always there.

Once we accept the First Noble Truth we begin to take the Buddha's advice seriously. The more clearly we see how our usual attempts to find happiness don't work, the more likely we are to take the prescription he offered. This is the premise AA is built on: until we admit we have a problem, we won't do anything about it.

Like the reformed alcoholic, though, after honestly recognizing our situation we're confronted by some daunting realities and the real work. It's obvious that facing and changing our undercurrent of unhappiness is going to be a big job; it's not a hobby we can restrict to weekends and holidays. Yet no matter how daunting the task, we also see that we don't have much choice. Since existential discomfort is happening this very moment, we must tend to it this very moment. It's not a problem to deal with "someday."

CHAPTER 3

THE CAUSE AND CURE IN A NUTSHELL

Human beings have this wonderful opportunity because of suffering. Instead of constantly resisting dissatisfaction, trying to sweep it under the carpet or lament and grieve about it and be pained by it, we should be grateful for it. It's our very best teacher.

—Ayya Khema
Being Nobody, Going Nowhere

If you check in with yourself enough, at some point you'll notice you're pretty darn content. When this happens, take an internal inventory. Do this several times, in a variety of situations, whenever you feel content, and eventually you'll notice a common denominator; what's missing is the desire for things to be different. Take, for instance, that golden moment during the delightful dinner party; though the conversation may have been good and the friends charming, the real reason you felt so content was that you essentially didn't want to change anything about where you were and what you were doing (any touch of dissatisfaction came from knowing the feeling would eventually end). That deep glow could have happened with different friends or while you were alone appreciating sunlight reflect off distant hills. The details don't matter, but the *not* wanting to change anything part does. This lack of wanting is the road to peacefulness.

It's simple really: when we want something—anything—to be other than the way it is right now, by definition things aren't right. We feel incomplete, without. The word the Buddha used for this longing, this perpetual itch, is "thirst," but it has also been called craving or desire. This craving takes a variety of forms, including ones we don't normally associate with desire, such as not wanting pain or not wanting to hear ideas we disagree with. It's an impulse underwritten and reinforced by selfishness (I want; I don't want; I want; I don't want). But no matter what we call it and no matter what the cause, to crave—to want and to not want—is to suffer. Dissatisfaction goes with desire, like wet with water. It cannot be otherwise.

Not realizing that what we really want is an absence of desire, we thrash about, looking here and there to satisfy our hungers. *Truly* end our thirst, even for a moment (which takes an instant of great purity), and we get a taste of nirvana. Totally end it forever, and we're completely enlightened.

How come we keep missing this? Wanting = unhappiness is a very easy formula to understand; you'd think every child would learn it before kindergarten. While the full explanation of our "essential oversight" will unfold over the course of this book, what follows here is a quick overview of the basics.

First, when we want something, in that very moment we're turning away from what we're actually doing and experiencing. After all, we are trying to escape things as they are. As a result, we're caught in a psychic catch-22: when unhappy, we *want* something to make us feel better, not realizing that the very remedy we're reaching for not only doesn't satisfy us, but makes us even more unhappy. Since the "medicine" we're taking makes us

sicker, we get more desperate and reach for even more medicine. We stay stuck in a circle of craving, more thirsty than ever.

We're so used to thinking we must get something or go
somewhere to feel good, that we have trouble even conceiving
that happiness comes from what is not. We turn happiness into
yet another thing to want. Many of us are apt to think of enlightenment or nirvana, the ultimate happiness, as a really positive
state of mind; one we need to *find*, as if it were a resort we could
check into. But actually, we're told, nirvana is experienced only
when craving and all negative states of mind are totally gone.
Peacefulness comes when the burning inside us stops. In other
words, when we genuinely trust the universe, when we don't
need or ask anything from it, we get what we truly want.

Probably the single biggest reason we miss the connection
between desire and dissatisfaction is we confuse pleasure with
happiness. It's an understandable mistake to make: when we're
content we feel good and when we feel pleasure we tend to be
somewhat content. But the two are different, and this explains
why a life spent seeking pleasure doesn't bring a life filled with
happiness. This doesn't suggest that Buddhism is against pleasure (a common misunderstanding, which will be discussed in
detail in chapter 13), only that pursuing pleasure is a dead-end
route to happiness.

Pleasure has two strikes against it as a source of happiness. First, "*somewhat* content" also means partially discontent.
And while a mostly favorable mix might not sound so bad, it's
not much to settle for when we remember that: a) when we feel
pleasure it quickly turns to grasping and longing—which makes
us discontent—and b) pleasant feelings are very temporary; we
have little control over its coming and going. In fact, when you
track 'em, you'll find pleasant sensations are downright mis-
chievous buggers, seemingly with a mind all their own.

If you doubt this, see if you can fill yourself with pleasure on command, and if you can, see how long it lasts. Maybe

we can muster a little pleasure whenever we want by thinking about some triumph or fantasy, but it's unlikely you'll get more than a few moments of feeling nice or feel anything approaching joy—unless you're already in a great mood. And then consider why you're in a great mood: you got a raise, you heard from a long lost friend, your team won a big game, etc. None of these things are in your control; all of them could have gone otherwise. No one, not even the Buddha, can count on always having pleasant sensations, but he did always have peace of mind.

The distinction between pleasure and happiness can be seen by looking at what happens when we're offered a hot fudge sundae while on a diet. As long as we hunger for the dessert, we'll feel unfulfilled. If we can't stand that desire anymore and decide to dig in, part of the satisfaction, especially during the first few bites, comes from being released, if briefly, from that acute pain of desire. Sometime after the first spoonfuls, though, the sundae may give little pleasure, or it may even turn on us ("it's too sweet").

Of course we might also feel pleasure in every bite. But what we don't usually notice is that while the dance of sugar and taste buds may cause pleasant sensations, the truly satisfying part comes from not wanting to be doing anything else in the world at that instant but sticking ice cream into our mouth. The contentment isn't coming from the taste itself—otherwise, we couldn't have different reactions to the sundae.

Distinguishing between pleasant feelings and satisfaction may sound like a philosophical splitting of hairs, but actually it's a very important and practical thing to notice. Since we can't always have pleasant sensations (eventually we'll finish the ice cream or get stuffed and then our pleasure and satisfaction will vanish, soon to be replaced by caloric regrets), it can't be a lasting or true source of happiness. But we can learn to always be accepting, to not want, and thus to be content.

DOING THE EIGHT-STEP

The obvious question then is, how can we learn *not* to crave, how can we learn to be content with the way things are right now, regardless of what that right now is? The Buddha's answer, his prescription for contentment, is traditionally known as the Eight-fold Noble Path. In a nutshell, this path works to free us from the three basic forms of craving—greed, hatred, and delusion—by cultivating their antidotes: equanimous awareness, compassion, and wisdom. Each "step" of the Eight-fold Path is associated with developing one of these three necessary, positive qualities: Three steps (right effort, right awareness, and right concentration) strengthen concentration or awareness; three steps (right speech, right action, and right livelihood) develop morality, and two steps (right thought and right understanding) help ripen our wisdom. Though I don't refer specifically to the eight steps in the balance of the pages ahead, this book is structured by the three essential aspects of the Eight-fold Path—concentration, ethics, and wisdom. Since this is book about a particular meditation technique, I've given most attention to the concentration aspect of the Eight-fold Path and tended to explore all three aspects of the path in relationship to the sensation-based vipassana technique. This doesn't imply that meditation alone is enough to free us from suffering.

Note also, that even though we may speak of compassion, awareness, and wisdom as three separate qualities, ultimately, they can't truly be distinguished from each other. To be fully compassionate, for example, requires the wisdom of knowing that there really isn't a "me" separate from everyone and everything else. It demands having a moment-to-moment presence of mind. Conversely, we can't be truly aware, insightful, or have peace of mind if we're filled with anger or hatred. Recognizing all this in a deep experiential way is true wisdom. To be wise is to be intimate with truth. So you could also call the Buddha's way truthfulness training.

Different schools of Buddhism have emphasized either loving-kindness, mindfulness, or insight in their practice, but since all lead to the same place and reinforce each other, they are all important to cultivate. This is why the Buddha's teachings are often symbolized by a wheel with eight spokes. Each spoke is equally important and all are connected in the center to compassion, awareness, and wisdom.

For a wheel to roll well, all its spokes must not only be strong, but of equal strength to the others. No aspect of Buddhist training should be sacrificed at the expense of another. So while each of the eight spokes is traditionally preceded by the word "right," what is really meant is "skillful." This suggests that while the Buddha gave us the basic recipe for happiness, we can't expect to find contentment simply by following a formula.

Some people object to the idea of training or using a method to find happiness. They believe happiness should just happen spontaneously. While this sounds nice and for a few it may even work (though according to the Buddha's teaching this would be the result of efforts made in this or a previous life), it won't work for most of us; we have too many negative, happiness-interfering tendencies. Only when we're freed from those obstructions can we become "spontaneously" happy. Once all our hindrances are gone, however, we can discard all methods. The Buddha referred to his teachings as a raft that can be left behind once we reach the other shore.

Everyone knows that to develop skill in any pursuit, we must work hard, learn from mentors, be disciplined, and stick to it. Whether we hope to become an ace golfer, a master artist, or a virtuoso pianist, we understand the key is practice, practice, practice under the guidance of a teacher. So why should finding happiness be different? And what could be a higher, more worthwhile "art" than happiness? Even if we set out concerned only about our own contentment, we'll find it won't really work unless we leave selfishness behind. In the end, everyone wins.

PART 2

CONCENTRATION:
STRENGTH OF MIND

The technique of whole-body vipassana involves three essential ingredients: sensations, awareness, and equanimity. As with creating a fine meal from a recipe, to do this practice well it's best if each key ingredient is not just included, but understood. So before beginning the meditating instructions, it's helpful to know why we focus on sensations throughout the body and why it's important to be aware and equanimous of our feelings.

After learning the instructions, it's worth considering if this method is how the Buddha himself meditated and recommended others do too. While the Buddha discouraged a cult of personality and this method would be just as effective whether it had his stamp of approval or not, by evaluating whether this technique is indeed his original method, we get an even more refined sense of why it works so well. Also, if you believe that, yes, this is most likely how the Buddha wanted us to meditate, you'll have more confidence to try it and stick with it.

CHAPTER 4

WHY SENSATION-BASED VIPASSANA
WORKS SO WELL

The institute in which I was studying hosted an insight medita-
tion (vipassana) retreat led by U Goenka, the well-known Indian
teacher from the Burmese tradition of U Ba Khin. The method of
meditation taught by Goenka is a highly effective technique of
developing concentrated mindfulness of body-sensations and feel-
ings, viewed in their aspects of being impermanent, unsatisfactory,
selfless. This retreat had an overwhelming impact on me. Within
the short period of ten days my consciousness was unquestionably
altered, and I gained direct experiential insights into the meaning
of the Buddhist teachings unlike anything I had ever realized
through the methods taught by my Tibetan teachers.
    —*Stephen Batchelor, author of*
    Buddhism Without Beliefs, in The Faith to Doubt

S
ince meditation can lead to an understanding where
words don't apply, some have shrouded the practice with
a mystique of holiness. This is understandable since meditation is a sacred pursuit, but it is also a practical one. The
Buddha maintained that what he taught was the truth of unhappiness and how to end it. Ultimately, meditation is a tool, a
method for increasing wisdom and decreasing discontent. So
while evaluating the effectiveness of a meditation technique or
comparing it to other methods may initially seem a little crude,
it's important to know whether the tool you're using is a good

one. Avoiding comparisons for fear it might be impolite seems overly timid.

That said, comparisons should naturally be done with respect, acknowledging that by definition one can't fully understand all methods (it's hard enough to really know one). And that for whatever reasons, some techniques will fit one personality better than another. That means people will always have preferences, even if technically one way should work better than another. After trying several of the most popular forms of Buddhist meditation practiced in this country* and then discovering that sensation-based vipassana is much more effective, I'm convinced there are reasons why that's so, even if those reasons don't hold for everyone.

Q

UNITING CONCENTRATION
AND MINDFULNESS TECHNIQUES

Though not often discussed, there is a split of sorts in the meditating world—namely, between concentration and mindfulness techniques. The difference between the two is suggested in a vignette the spiritual teacher Krisnamurti once recounted after traveling in India. Krisnamurti was sitting in the front seat of a car next to a chauffeur. In the back, three of his students were intently discussing awareness. At one point, just as the back seat passengers asked Krisnamurti a question about awareness, the car happened to hit a goat, though the driver never stopped or

---

* I'm only superficially familiar with Tibetan Buddhism and its various practices. Consequently, I was very interested to read Stephen Batchelor's experience of S.N. Goenka's course (see quotation at the opening of this chapter). Curiously, though, after parting ways with the Tibetan teachings, Batchelor became a Zen monk in Korea. Apparently, he was drawn to the sense of doubt cultivated in some forms of Zen.

slowed the car. Those in the back seat were so absorbed by their conversation, they never even noticed the accident.

Concentration meditators typically focus on one thing at a time—a mantra, a candle's flame, counting breaths—to the exclusion of everything else. Those practicing mindfulness cultivate a choiceless awareness of whatever comes up. The two methods aren't exactly at odds. The Buddha made it clear that both concentration and awareness must be developed to achieve insight. And each technique involves aspects of the other; there isn't a thick line separating the two. Yet each method has a different emphasis and effect on its practitioners.

The distinction between the techniques can be seen in the two branches within Zen Buddhism: Rinzai and Soto. Rinzai Zen practitioners concentrate on a koan—a logically unanswerable question. The Rinzai Zen meditator attempts to stay focused on his koan until the thinking mind exhausts itself. Although the most famous koan is "What is the sound of one hand clapping?" what's actually practiced more is "doing MU." That is, repeating the word MU over and over, while focusing attention in the pit of your belly. (Technically, the koan is "What is MU?" which means "nothingness" or "void" in Japanese, but typically one focuses only on the last word.) Non-MU thoughts and feelings are ignored. This practice builds a mental power and focus that is important for cultivating calmness and the ability to stay present. Done whole-heartedly and relentlessly, concentrating like this can cause time, worries, pain, and thoughts to drop away, leaving the meditator in an expansive, tranquil, and wordless state.

The Soto Zen meditator, following the tradition established by its founder, master Dōgen, ostensibly has no agenda. One simply sits still, trying to be aware of whatever is happening in the moment—a bird singing, your breathing, the pain in your leg, the sound of your heartbeat. While this takes concentration too (otherwise you'd spend most of your time on the meditation cushion absorbed in daydreams or worries), the focus isn't single-pointed. Thoughts can even be fodder for mindfulness. What's important is maintaining an observing, nonattached state of mind. This type of awareness can evoke a gentle and calm openness, which makes it easier to accept life as it unfolds. It can bring the recognition that there is no "me," only ever-changing processes. Recognizing this undermines our grasping ego.

While both methods—concentration and mindfulness—can bring tranquility, each has strengths and drawbacks. Not surprisingly, one-pointed concentration makes it simpler to stay focused, which brings a strength and stability of mind. Achieve full absorption and you'll find a purity of consciousness that can loosen negative thought patterns even after the experience slips away. But a single-focus practice has a more closed, less receptive flavor than a mindfulness practice. To focus only on one thing, it's necessary to disregard, well, everything else, including whatever your body or emotions are expressing. This leaves our tendency to ignore and repress unwanted feelings intact. So at the unconscious level our mind doesn't change much.

In mindfulness practice there's nothing to push away, which gives one's awareness a softer, more investigative and curious quality. Our natural tendency to ignore unwanted feelings doesn't automatically disappear, but we're at least more likely to notice that habit operating. The downside to this technique is that it's generally harder to do without losing one's focus; we're more likely to get caught up in our thoughts and fantasies. This can interfere with developing the stillness and tranquility necessary for deeper insight.

The beauty of sensation-based vipassana is that it combines the best elements of both methods. Sensations, which are what you concentrate on as you move your attention throughout your body, provide a definite focus which fosters concentration, and the scanning patterns you follow (see chapter 8) give a tracking, are-you-with-the-program feedback mechanism, mak-

ing it easier to catch yourself when you drift. Yet, you're still cultivating a receptive attention. Sensitivity to sensations requires
being open to what is happening in the moment. We're simply
uncovering what is there, whether we want it to be or not.
Practicing properly demands that we remain aware of the full
range of our feelings, from subtle to overwhelming. In this way,
we're less likely to be distracted by our usual emotional defenses.
And we're more likely to stay engaged in the process, as our feelings hold more intrinsic interest than repeating a mantra or
phrase again and again.

What about concentrating on our breath—doesn't that
allow for a receptive, yet focused attention? It does; the breath
makes an excellent focus for meditation. It is always there, flowing in and out. By observing the *sensations* created by your
breath, you can develop an acute sensitivity. For this reason,
sensation-based vipassana meditators use their breath to establish concentration and as an anchor when they're feeling too
overwhelmed or distracted to focus on sensations. But once that
calmness is achieved, attention is turned to feelings throughout
the body so we can learn to accept all of our feelings, including
the most subtle.

It's worth noting that when you concentrate on your
breath, even if you think you're observing the breath itself, what
you're really noticing are the effects of your breath. Try breathing though your nose for a few moments and you'll see. Maybe
you'll notice a bit of wind whistling, but mainly we're aware of
our breath from its *touch* as it moves through our nasal passages
and beyond. To know it in another way you must visualize or
imagine it in some fashion, not just experience it as it is. So as
long as you concentrate on the sensations your breath creates,
it's still honing sensitivity to feelings.

And what about observing our thoughts? Certainly
thoughts are ephemeral, constantly changing and nearly always
available as something to focus on. Some vipassana traditions do

make use of thoughts as objects of meditation. One simply tries to observe their coming and going without getting absorbed by the "text" of the thoughts. The trouble is, as anyone who's tried this knows, it's exceedingly difficult to do. Thoughts tend to suck us into their drama. And as writer and meditation teacher Stephen Levine put it, "As long as we're identifying with content, we're not really free."

Naturally, difficulty shouldn't disqualify a meditation method—at least if it were more effective than others. After all, it's not as though any type of meditation is easy. Rather, it's the very nature of thought which makes it a problematic object of meditation. Thoughts tend to conceal the fundamental truths the Buddha is directing us to: namely impermanence, the inability of any experience to provide lasting satisfaction, and our belief in an unchanging permanent self. This will become clearer as we investigate the difference between sensations and thoughts a bit more.

THINKING ABOUT THINKING

In chapter 1, we observed that the difference between the concept "arm" and the experience of our arm is essentially the difference between a map and the place it charts. A map may come in handy at times, but we always know it's just a symbolic representation. We don't mistake it for being the world itself—as we do with our thoughts. Shifting from living mostly in our thoughts to being more experientially based is like going from being an armchair traveler to having an adventure.

Ideas define. They capture a thing or two, or at most, a few things at a time. Of course subtle and complex thinking is possible, but the very nature of a thought is to highlight a particular aspect of something and block out most everything else. Come up with a thought, any thought—whether it's "there's a fly on the ceiling" or "the global reach of large multinational corporations is changing the historic rules of national sovereignty"—and look at how it narrows focus. We're zeroing in on particulars, confining our attention in a way that, like blinders, restricts us somewhat. This narrowing is good for communicating or, if we're focused on the right things, for analysis. But it's bad for experiencing the reality of the moment directly.

The limitations of thought have many spiritually relevant consequences. Thoughts, for instance, tend to draw our attention away from what we're actually feeling. Conceptualizing dulls our awareness and senses. When we live in our thoughts we tend not to notice our actual experiences and instead end up inhabiting a world of familiar assumptions and stereotypes, notions that give our surroundings a sense of constancy and familiarity. No wonder our world can appear flat and boring, despite knowing it's not really that way.

As was also noted in chapter 1, since ideas have the effect of "freezing" the fleeting, ever-changing nature of reality, they give us a sense of solidity that isn't really there. We end up approaching our life as though it were a thing—as though a detailed obituary could capture our existence, or that if we could manage the distinct events/things that make up our life in just the right way, things would be just perfect (and then we could keep them that way).

Naturally my goal isn't to beat on ideas and thinking, particularly the analytic and introspective variety which can be valuable tools, and even used effectively for spiritual progress. Since ideas can work like a map, having good maps can help us get where we want to go. Still, at some point, the map must be put aside, or only consulted occasionally; the real work of any journey comes from the effort of moving ahead step-by-step, moment-by-moment.

Even clear thinking often creates problems for us. We tend to take our insights too literally, holding our perceptions as *con-*

clusions and turning the sharpness of a good thought into something that cuts the world into two (usually black and white). Transpersonal theorist Ken Wilber points out that, "Every boundary creates two warring opposites." It's no accident then that most of us easily fall into an us-and-them/right-and-wrong mentality which squeezes out subtlety, paradox, and shades of gray—just the place where the truth and mystery usually reside. As others have said, the rational mind is a good servant, but a bad master.

Of course, most of our thoughts couldn't actually be considered analytical or logical. Rather they're more like expressions of emotions that frame and color what we experience. Yet since most of us are unaware of that and we're unaware of the concretizing and narrowing aspect of our thoughts, we're captured by them without realizing it. Our emotion-thoughts spin a self-censored universe, framed by our ideas about how things are and should be. It's rare that we notice this since the very nature of thoughts is to create a sense of certainty and solidity.

A thought can expose the restrictive aspect of ideas in general, noting their tendency to inhibit genuine freedom, but if we *only* think about that without having extensive wordless experiences, it's as though we've just moved from one room to another. Philosophizing alone can never truly allow us to escape the quasi-fictional world we create. Since our thoughts act like sunglasses and we rarely, if ever, take off the tinted lenses, it's very hard to recognize that we're even wearing them.

By focusing directly and completely on sensations, we're able to have experiences without frames and solidity. An uninterpreted sensation is an experience without any conclusions or boundaries. Unlike a thought/statement (any thought or statement) which makes the implied claim that "this is the way things are," a sensation doesn't declare anything; it simply is what is, allowing us to experience a basic, if momentary, truth. As Matthew Flickstein points out in *Journey to the Center*, all thoughts have time and space as a reference point, so we tend to be pinned down to a spot and oriented toward the past or future. Yet reality itself—insight into the true nature of our experience—can only happen in the present and can't be captured by words.

There is another, crucial reason that sensations are the focus of meditation: they are what we actually react to. As will be detailed more in the next chapter, every thought we have is accompanied by a sensation (though not necessarily vice versa) and it's the feeling aspect of that combination that moves us. Every thought or emotion we have is meaningful not because of it's inherent logic, poetry, or injustice, but because of how it makes us feel.

Focusing on sensations puts us more directly in touch with what's motivating us, while at the same time helping to free us from the storylines which tend to obscure our feelings. In this way, greater awareness to our sensations increases our emotional sensitivity. While most of us can't help but be aware of extreme emotions, the thought side of an emotion often disguises or obscures our feelings so that we misinterpret what's really bothering us or completely missing our more subtle feelings.

Awareness of our actual feelings adds depth and texture to our life as well as providing an avenue for changing habitual reactions. To truly change and purify our minds at the deepest level we must know what we're feeling at our depths. So no matter what we tell ourselves—"it's okay," "just let go," "no worries"—if we're not aware and truly accepting of any feeling aspect associated with that thought, we'll still react to that thought/feeling. By paying attention to sensations, we can catch everything that irks and tantalizes us, which helps keep us honest in a way we usually aren't.

So much of our psychic activity is in service of creating pleasant feelings or distracting ourselves from painful ones that we miss how our feelings are shaping our thoughts. Then, the defining-concretizing aspect of thoughts which often accompanies our feelings blinds us to what is really going on, holding negative mental patterns in place. When we focus on our sensations and loosen the grip of our thoughts, lots of territory can open up, revealing just how big our mind really is. At that point, even if feelings/thoughts arise that would usually make us anxious, it doesn't grab hold of us in the same way. Our fears can float by, acknowledged, yet without shutting us down.

To some extent, every type of meditation reveals that we are master self-deceivers, but by tending to sensations it's harder to be tricked since we experience our feelings directly. Since the body and mind aren't separate, by scanning our body, we're also scanning our whole mind. By observing every piece of our body, inside and out, we're bringing awareness to what might otherwise have remained in dark or buried corners of our mind. Think of letting sunlight into a basement: once you can see what's down there, it won't be so scary. And any mold that was growing (in the psyche's case, that would be defenses and the complexes formed around them) can naturally begin to dissolve. To quote the Buddhist therapist Mark Epstein again, "What is ultimately therapeutic for many people is not so much the narrative construction of their past to explain their suffering, but the direct experience . . . of the emotions, emotional thoughts, or physical remnants of emotional thoughts with which they are stuck."

With sensation-based vipassana, the act of meditating can be simultaneously therapeutic, calming, and enlightening.

CHAPTER 5

RECONSIDERING OUR BODY

The body holds the mind just as the mind contains the body.
Deep feelings of loss and pain are recorded in the tissues of the
body as well as in the mind. In deep quietude, the mind can free
the body of its holding, just as in deep grounding and surrender
the body can unlock the deepest secrets of the mind.
—Stephen Levine, A Gradual Awakening

Most of us have a curious relationship with our body. We exercise, pluck out unwanted hairs, take vitamins, and check the mirror throughout the day. We buy high-tech mattresses to sooth an aching back, get a massage when our neck is stiff, and maybe even take a yoga class. Yet despite all the attention, we don't really *listen* to our body. We tend to use our body, treating it as if it were simply a complicated machine that we owned. Naturally we hope, even pray, this machine doesn't break down, but we still experience our body from a distance. Even those who consider their body their temple usually regard it as a separate, if sophisticated, building to be well maintained for its resident (thinking of it as "my body" in a *roughly* similar vein that we think of "my car"). We may appreciate the body's mechanical intelligence, but its real intelligence, its sensitivity, and wisdom is overlooked. Even spiritual teachers often miss the importance of being sensitive to feelings throughout our body, reinforcing the mind-body schism.

As medical research is revealing, our body is more than housing for its occupant: it's an integral expression of who we are. Our body mirrors our mind and our mind reflects our body. As the pioneering biochemist Candace Pert put it, "The body is the actual manifestation, in physical space, of the mind."

Usually, when we seek self-knowledge, we mine our thoughts, or think about what we're feeling. Yet, having done that countless times, you may have noticed a couple of unnerving things about the relationship between your thoughts and the truth: first, you can't always believe what comes out of your own mouth, and second you can't even always trust what you think. Our capacity and creativity for psychological avoidance, rationalization, and self-deception is awesome. Even the sharpest intellects are often way off when it comes to insight into their own psyche and motivations. In fact, sometimes the more clever you are, the more ingenious your rationalizations are.

But your body doesn't lie. When you're defeated, it hunches; when you're happy, it beams. If you pay close attention, you'll notice that many of the itches, aches, pains, and tics we have throughout a day express unpleasant feelings or distract us from unwelcome emotions. And of course any time you blush, become shaky from stage fright, or break into a nervous, cold sweat you can plainly see that the body reveals what you're feeling. How else, after all, could lie detectors work?

In a way, it's silly to point out that our body expresses our emotions since we already intuitively know it. When someone frowns or squirms in their chair, there's no doubt what they're feeling. Likewise, we recognize crying, belly laughs, and animated gestures as a "soul" bubbling over. But while we readily interpret and react to such passions, we miss a basic and significant fact about them: emotions are embodied; our feelings are literally felt. If they weren't, we would be like robots. Emotions would simply be electrical impulses, not alive, meaningful events. It's no accident that the word "feeling" is used both for an emotional and tactile experience. It's also no coincidence that our language is filled with expressions such as "pain in the neck," "getting it off my chest," "having cold feet," and "can't stomach it." Or, when somebody has lost their humanity—whether a psychopath or ruthless CEO—we say he is heartless and has no feelings.

Research on neuropeptides, the molecules of our emotions (discussed in more detail in chapter 11), confirms that we truly do feel emotions throughout our body. While our gray matter is our primary analyzer and "thinker," our mind isn't located only in our brain. Neuropeptides and their receptors, the communicators of emotions that are so abundant in the brain, are found *everywhere* in our body. Our mind is not a command central operation but more like an information-processing field. Every cell in our body is capable of feeling; every cell can experience emotion. A gut instinct isn't just an expression, it's an emotional reaction that hasn't been translated into words. Once we think about it, we realize it couldn't be otherwise. If we didn't have some degree of consciousness throughout our body, how could we experience sensations *everywhere* on us?

After recognizing that feelings by definition are felt in the body, it becomes clearer how emotional disease can so often turn into physical disease—a fact that has been documented by volumes of research showing the connection between our emotions, illness, and healing. Of course it's not that getting angry or having a bad day will ruin your liver; unpleasant feelings are an unavoidable part of life, and consciously experiencing them is healthy. Rather, it's being unaware of our anger and distress and consistently repressing them and trying to keep them at bay that takes its toll. Neuroscientists have learned that there is multidirectional intercellular communication throughout the brain and body. When we try to deny or block what we're feeling, we restrict the biological information flow to an area (or areas) of our body. Naturally this stresses those organs affected by the freeze-out, making them more prone to illness. In this way, blindness to our feelings has physical as well as psychological costs.

When we're attuned to our actual feelings, we're less likely to misinterpret what our body is telling us. Usually, when we have a headache, back pain, heartburn, rash, or allergy, we reach for a pill or call the doctor, chiropractor, or naturopath. Of course sometimes that's the smartest thing to do, but often those maladies are simply signs of neglected emotions or indications that we need to attend more closely to what we're feeling. Once we do that, the pain frequently disappears without any outside help. Before practicing vipassana, S.N. Goenka had severe migraines that sent him seeking help from doctors and hospitals throughout the world. Nothing worked medically and he was in danger of turning into an opium addict. Not long after doing this type of meditation, however, the headaches disappeared. For myself, after meditating this way for a few months, a rash I'd had since college disappeared and allergies I had for almost a decade went away (except for an occasional and mild stuffed nose in the fall). While one shouldn't begin meditating to cure an ailment, good health is often a pleasant side effect.

The reason the body affects the mind, and the mind the body, is that the two aren't just related or "connected," as the open-minded medical community now recognizes, they're essentially inseparable—two sides of one coin. The biochemical occurrence of a thought or feeling is simultaneously both that ungraspable and ephemeral experience and a "physical" event.

Fear, for example, can be described both as a feeling/thought and in terms of adrenaline hormone molecules. Our thoughts and experiences could be expressed either as an affective state or in chemical terms.

Perhaps the best and most dramatic evidence indicating the inseparability of mind and body shows up in people with multiple personality disorders. Within the same individual body, different personalities exhibit different physiologies. One personality, for example, may have diabetes, yet when that persona disappears, so does the insulin deficiency. In other cases, warts, scars, rashes, allergies, and epilepsy come and go depending upon which personality is in force. In instances where a childlike persona emerges, she requires smaller dosages of medicine than the adult personalities. This extreme malleability challenges our usual notions of identity, definition, and the relationship between the material and spiritual.

For most of us, the nondualistic idea that the mind and body are two simultaneous expressions of the mindbody (or bodymind, if you prefer) is difficult to grasp. We're so thought-identified that we tend to think that "Brains 'R' Us" (as though the brain wasn't part of the body). In recent years, Descartes has taken a lot of heat from mindbody integrators for his influential "I think; therefore I am," but he's got lots of company, past and present. For most of us, our thoughts are *me*. Our ego, our sense that we are in control (damn it!) holds tight to that illusion. Also, the focus-on-one-thing-at-a-time aspect of a concept causes us to stumble on a concurrent truth. Like those ambiguous illustrations in intro to psychology books, which show a drawing that can be seen either as a vase or two profiles, we have trouble holding both as true at the same time. Our mind flips back and forth between the two interpretations, but we want to settle on one or the other.

So when we stub our toe and it hurts, we think of it as a body event—even though our mind obviously is participating/affected by the experience as well. And when we're depressed, we think of it as a mental experience—even though it's accompanied by biochemical changes such as sinking hormone levels, desensitized neuropeptide receptors, and a tendency for blood platelet cells to clump. The tears from a depressed cry even have different traces of chemicals than tears of joy. (Not surprisingly, the chronically depressed are four times more likely to get sick than the average person.) Of course, there's no reason why we can't look at or speak of just one "side" of the mindbody, but we miss the real picture if we forget that what happens to one simultaneously affects the other. What's important to remember for understanding why sensation-based vipassana is so effective is that every thought and emotion we have has correlated sensations—even if we're not aware of it at the time.

OUR BODY "HOLDS" OUR UNCONSCIOUS

As it turns out, ignorance is not bliss. Even when we're not consciously aware of our feelings, we still react to them. Those reactions then don't simply vanish, but leave a residue of tension. That tension then accumulates and is held in our body. And those accumulated unacknowledged feelings essentially create our unconscious.

Toward the end of his life, Freud theorized that our unconscious is carried in the soma, or body. Most of us, however, still think of it as residing somewhere in our brain, inseparable from our thoughts. So it's worth briefly considering why our unconscious processes should be largely sensation- and body-based (though not disconnected from our brain or, often, from our thoughts). The reason, it seems, is a legacy of our evolution as a species.

As evolutionary theory tells us, we are adapted from simpler animals whose ability to think was rudimentary at best.

Keeping that in mind, it makes sense that our mind-body should be built around processing sensations. For example, when an ant's eyes and feelers transmit information to the rest of its body, it doesn't say, "Hey, cupcake crumb to the left." Instead, sensations announcing that news must run through its body. Likewise, details relevant to a frog, rabbit, or bear's survival must be processed mostly via sensations and instinctive reactions.

By developing the ability to think and be self-aware, our essentially sensation-based orientation wasn't lost; the two just developed in concert with each other. Having conscious and unconscious—or mind- and body-centered—capacities actually offers all sorts of practical advantages. While one part of us is figuring and analyzing, another can make sure that our arms and legs are behaving themselves and we don't fall into a ditch.

As data from our senses, sensations allow us to keep tabs on what's going on in our immediate environment. In this way, sensations act as a kind of mood music, usually in the background and unnoticed, but still letting us know what the general atmosphere is. If any threats or treats come our way, say a stalking tiger or an enticing potential mate appears, the rhythm, beat, and volume of our feelings change significantly, grabbing our full attention. This functional aspect of our unconscious ability to process sensation becomes more obvious when we sleep. While the thinking guys shut down for the night, we're still able to shift positions, swat away mosquitoes, know if we need an urgent visit to the toilette, and respond to alarming noises.

Of course our nightly unconscious activities are better known for bringing us dreams than for allowing us to toss and turn. At first glance, dreaming seems like a purely thought-centric affair, but actually our nightly adventures (like every thought we have) are accompanied by feelings too. That thoughts should have a feeling component also makes sense as a design feature: we need to intuitively know whether what we're thinking or experiencing is helpful or problematic. Feelings of pleasure and pain associated with thoughts and emotions help us remember which experiences we want to repeat and which to avoid. As neuroscientist Joseph LeDoux points out in *The Emotional Brain*, while we can have feelings without thoughts, we can't have a thought without a feeling.

As a practical setup, our conscious/unconscious arrangement works well, but there is a downside: although we are essentially moved by sensations and emotions, except for strong feelings, we're naturally set up to be only marginally aware of them. And, when feelings become so strong we can't help but notice, they tend to have such a strong grip on us that we're at their whim.

The attempt to bring greater awareness to the veiled motives and feelings driving us is where Buddhism overlaps with psychotherapy. The two tend to diverge, however, in how to handle the feelings that arise, especially in the way a meditator brings detailed and nonreactive attention to their sensations.

CHAPTER 6

DEFROSTING DETACHMENT

---

*Suffering never befalls him who clings not to mind and body
and is detached.*
—*The Buddha*

*Most of us suffer through our dark emotions or grab at
pleasant ones—like prizes at a county fair—but we aren't
able to maintain our focus or our equilibrium around the
emotions. Being creative means experiencing emotions with
consciousness and skill.*
—*Karla McLaren,* Emotional Genius

The very idea of detachment makes most Westerners uncomfortable. At worst, we think of sociopaths who cheat and maim without remorse, or catatonics who barely function. At best, we picture Clint Eastwood staring down a gang of desperadoes, or Walt "Clyde" Frazier sinking a game winning jumper and showing only a hint of a smile. Somewhere in-between these archetypes is an impassive statue of the Buddha or a loin-clothed ascetic, lying on that fabled bed of nails (which mostly seem to exist in *New Yorker* cartoons during the fifties). The yogi's talent seems great for inclement weather, but these impassive sorts don't seem quite human. We assume they just must know how to zone out really well. As psychotherapist, author, and vipassana teacher Dr. Paul Fleischman put it, "Most people believe being detached means having a flat affect." Hardly something to aspire to.

Jack Engler, another therapist-writer-meditation teacher, once assumed that too. Not long after he started meditating, he told his teacher that the way he saw it, the outcome of extensive meditation training sounded pretty dull. He imagined transcending pain and pleasure meant entering a numbing, non-feeling existence. "Once you get rid of desire and aversion," he asked his teacher, "where's the chutzpah? The pizzazz? The juice? Life would be pretty tepid and uninteresting if you didn't enjoy anything at all."

Engler's teacher laughed and said, "You don't understand. Life is so much more full of zest now than it was when I was carrying all that baggage around. Now each experience has its own taste. And then it passes and it's gone. And then the next experience has its own taste." Like many of us, Engler had confused pleasure with contentment and reaction with interest.

Since we're usually not familiar with experiencing sensations without reacting to them, it's easy to be confused by detachment—even if we decide we're "for it." Before learning full-body vipassana, I misunderstood and struggled with detachment. I knew equanimity was an important part of the Buddhist path; I liked the idea of being unflappable; I read and reread the famous line of the third Zen patriarch, Sengstan: "The Great Way is not difficult for those who have no preferences." But actually doing that (especially off the meditating cushion), was a different story, and rarely satisfying. My attempts at detachment were generally stiff efforts to harden myself against things that made me uncomfortable. I didn't have the experiential vocabulary to just be, so I imagined what I *should* be like and got all bollixed up when my reactions didn't fit that scenario.

After years of trying this confused type of detachment, I unofficially conceded it wasn't working for me and sort of pretended that detachment wasn't part of Buddhism—or only so when I meditated. Off the cushion, I tried focusing on being-here-now and maintaining an open mind (not consciously realizing that an open mind is an expression of a detached mind).

But detachment is an important part of Buddhism. In fact, it's one of the few cornerstones that all the Buddhist traditions agree on. Whether it's Theravada, Mahayana, or Vajrayana, they tell us the road to liberation comes from not holding on to anything. Reading the ancient texts, one finds again and again the counsel to be detached. Many of these translations, however, can sound old fashioned, stiff, and severe. So somehow I only partially heard their advice. Naturally, vaguely associating detachment with zombies, the emotionally dead, or superheroes didn't help either.

No doubt I have a thicker skull than most, but it wasn't until I started practicing full-body vipassana that I discovered the problem wasn't with detachment, but how I understood it. I wasn't being equanimous, but dissociating (which is actually what happens to psychopaths, hardened bureaucrats, and anyone who is unfeeling). After learning to focus on the sensations in my body, it became clear that true nonattachment is only possible if you're very much aware of what you're actually feeling. Otherwise, you're trying to avoid the truth of the moment—which is repression

I had been trying to think or will my way to detachment, and that doesn't work; for not only did I get caught by what was irritating me, but I also got snagged by the idea that things shouldn't be bothering me. Much better is to just be with whatever is happening (expecting that most of the time it's not going to be what we fancy). Taking this tact is the difference between fighting against the wind and floating with it. Even if you're not wafting on a gentle tropical breeze, you're still not struggling.

It finally sunk in that what's really meant by detachment is complete acceptance. Once I substituted the word "acceptance" for "detachment" and even for "equanimity," which S.N. Goenka so often uses, it became much easier to be equanimous. "Equanimity" is an excellent word to express the balanced, serene, and unfettered state of mind meditation tries to cultivate, and it doesn't have the negative associations of "detachment," but for many Westerners, it too lacks a certain warmth. Likewise for "nongrasping" or "nonclinging," which also accurately describe what one is after. Yet it's hard to feel inspired by a "non."

"Acceptance" has a gentleness and kindness to it that feels right. When you're truly accepting, you're both completely available and able to feel deeply. You're allowing the universe to unfold as it will. Since you're okay with whatever happens, you are equanimous. To accept is to trust; to trust is to relax. Only when we have nothing to protect can we let go and be peaceful. In this way, acceptance, nongrasping, detachment—whatever you want to call it—is necessary for genuine freedom.

Acceptance, unlike detachment, also has deep western spiritual roots. Jesus on the cross, compassionate even to his tormentors, is a paradigm of acceptance we can aspire to—even if that kind of tranquility seems beyond most of us. More accessible is the Serenity Prayer: "May I have the serenity to accept the things I cannot change, the courage to change the things I can, and the wisdom to know the difference." Or the Talmud's, "the rich man is content with his lot."

Yet perhaps "acceptance" isn't the perfect word either. It's exactly what we need to do when we're struggling and experiencing difficult feelings, but when things are going well, our efforts to be accepting readily slip into grasping. Being accepting, opening to whatever is, tends to feel good (even in the midst of "unpleasant feelings"), and as the pleasant feelings associated with that softening kick in, we easily get attached to them, wanting them to never leave. When this happens, we're no longer content with just the way things are. And that is what we're really after: a mind so relaxed and contented that nothing needs to be changed. While equanimity or serenity may initially sound cold or unfeeling to some; think of their opposites: agitation, uneasiness, discontentment, anxiousness. Why would we ever want those? But every time we stray from equanimity, that's where we end up in some form.

Equanimity has another big benefit: it helps us see the truth more clearly. An equanimous or balanced mind is an objective one. True insight comes from observing only what is and nothing more. In this way, equanimity is the antidote to our usual, powerful inclination to see what we like and already believe. To experience ultimate truth, one must be free of all distortions. It means being aligned, body and mind, with the truth.

We can get some sense, in material terms, of the strength and mastery that comes from objectivity by looking at the scientific community's accomplishments (however imperfect their attempts at impartiality may be at times). By insisting on rigorous objective standards, the scientific method has yielded impressive knowledge and technological prowess. When that objectivity is missing in us (and vipassana meditation is designed to develop it), so is our ability to cut through our fog of rationalizations, confusion, and misperception—our own biases. If we never sought objectivity and simply believed things are the way they seem, let's face it, most of us would still think the earth is flat and the center of the universe.

While the above focus on phrasing may appear to have digressed into a sloppy William Safire "On Language" column, my point isn't linguistic nitpicking. The exact word or words one chooses doesn't matter. In fact, it seems that there isn't a single perfect word to convey the state of unhindered serenity the Buddha wanted us to develop. But clarity does matter. Equanimity is the goal of this form of meditation (which doesn't imply cultivating other positive mind states, such as loving kindness aren't also crucial) and understanding what that means is important, especially since we've grown up in a culture unfamiliar or even antagonistic to the idea. The important thing to remember about cultivating equanimity is that you want to be objective without losing a yielding sense of softness. You want to feel completely relaxed, but without getting so cozy you don't want to acknowledge disorienting or difficult feelings.

THE IRONIES OF THE MISUNDERSTOOD BUDDHA

There are a couple ironies associated with the West's misunderstanding and projection of a detached, unfeeling Buddha. Done skillfully, equanimity gives one more space to have a rich emotional life, feel more deeply, and have greater empathy. When we're not overpowered by our feelings, we can experience them directly and with greater nuance; we learn to accept our emotional life in all its guises; and we have more room for letting in another's hardships.

In *Emotional Intelligence*, Daniel Goleman cites a university study on emotional reactions which indicates people generally fall into one of two camps: those who distance themselves from strong emotions and those who get swamped by them. To illustrate, he gave examples of the two extremes. One fellow was so numb that after noticing his dorm was on fire, without any sense of urgency, he causally walked to get a fire extinguisher and doused the flames. On the other extreme was a woman who was "distraught for days" after losing her favorite pen.* While the reactions of the catatonic guy and the panicky gal are so dif-

---

* Research shows that men tend to distance themselves from their emotions while women tend to feel both positive and negative emotions more powerfully, making it more likely that uncomfortable feelings will overwhelm them.

ferent they may initially seem to have little in common, both are unable to handle their feelings. As psychotherapist Mark Epstein put it in *Thoughts Without a Thinker*: "When we refuse to acknowledge the presence of unwanted their feelings, we are as bound to them as when we give ourselves over to them, indignantly and self-righteously."

Contrary to popular belief, getting your emotions off your chest—say, yelling at someone who is annoying you—isn't a healthy (or productive) way to process your frustration. Without at least some measure of equanimity, focusing on our emotions tends to make us roil in them. Who hasn't worked themselves into a frenzy thinking about someone who's done us wrong? That kind of reaction only strengthens our distress without helping us work through it. Any decent therapist will tell you the key to good communication is empathy and not becoming overly reactive. That doesn't imply we should stifle feelings or not freely acknowledge them, since those would only suppress them, but it does indicate two crucial points: one, at least some measure of objectivity is needed to skillfully handle our feelings; two, feeding negative states of mind with more negativity only creates more problems.

It's also ironic that a detached Buddha is imagined to be aloof and out of touch when actually it is our attachments—our judgments, beliefs, self-centeredness, and attempts to control things—that deceive us and distance us from others.

To appreciate how our preferences and beliefs influence even what we call "facts," consider, from a neurological perspective, how we see. Our eye isn't just a camera taking pictures "out there" without editorializing. Neuroscientists tell us that in order for something to even be registered as "seen," the electrical impulses that hit our retina must interact both with the cortex (the part of the brain where "thinking" and interpretation take place) and the limbic system (or the emotional/motivational part of the brain). For each neuropathway that connects from the retina to the thalamus (a kind of relay station in the brain for transmitting emotional, cognitive, and instinctual impulses), there are more than eighty times as many fibers communicating information to that same point *from* the cortex. It's estimated that only twenty percent of what we see comes from unadorned data that the retina has absorbed; the rest comes from information added by other parts of the brain. In other words, typically, eighty percent of what we see is a projection influenced by our feelings and thoughts. Apparently, most of our brain cells are never directly affected by the "outside" world.

This eighty percent-added piece of even "simple" vision explains how the same person—even a stranger—can evoke different reactions in different people. Our emotional cargo and interpretative filters are bathing that perception in our own light. Clearly, the fewer presumptions we make, the fewer biases we have, the more accurate our "vision." And when we remember that much of our emotions and "thinking" are underwritten by instinctual impulses and desires, then we recognize that the interference isn't just a little tinting, but more like a glare.

We get the full-blown effect of this "background" interference after we fall asleep. Once we lose direct contact with outside stimulus, elaborate dream worlds emerge. Our mind freely spins its web. What most of us don't realize, however, is that this spinning doesn't stop even after we get out of bed, it's just kept in check by the twenty percent of reality we bump up against. Equanimity can act as a corrective to our usual distorting preconceptions.

Since most of us don't notice our misconceptions, we rarely notice how they keep us in our own world. Self-centered outlooks and righteous convictions create barriers between ourselves and others. In situations more charged than a stranger's face, it's easy to see how this works: a misunderstanding produces different, seemingly irreconcilable, versions of what happened and who was "right." Of course, some differences are legitimate, but the heat and frustration that often accompany those differences are fueled by each of us living in our own ego-colored, my-version-must-be-right cosmos.

$$\mathbb{Q}$$

NOT JUST FOR SPIRITUAL OLYMPIANS

To lose or at least lessen these self-obstructions we don't need to be a Tibetan meditation master. When we listen to someone else without an agenda, without any expectations, we both notice the difference. Our presence is truly felt and a real connection is made. Likewise, we feel the difference when someone listens to us without trying to change us and without laying in wait so they can make their point. Such openness is the manifestation of an accepting and nongrasping mind. Meditation helps us develop this further, but the quality isn't something exotic or strange; it's a capacity we all have. If we didn't, we could never develop it further.

This openness or acceptance is at the heart of what makes meditation relaxing. It's what inspires all those stress-reduction classes at the Y. Experiments on meditators confirm that meditation can indeed be calming: while on the cushion, one's heart rate and breathing tend to slow down, reducing the need for oxygen, and brainwave patterns shift to alpha-waves, which indicate a healing, relaxed-state. These come with being more accepting.

When we're not accepting, when we try to force things to go our way, ironically, we only stymie what we're *really* looking for from the thing we're trying to get: contentment. We seem to forget that our influence on events is limited; things usually don't turn out as planned (and rarely *just* as we want). I've yet to meet anyone who's gotten *all* their wishes met for a whole day, let alone a week. Nor have I met anyone who has trained their friends or family, including their children, to act just the way they want them to. Even dictators have limited success with this. Drop the whole effort to control, though, accept whatever comes your way, and paradoxically you're granted a happiness that's like having infinite control.

When we rely on any thing for our happiness, we're always vulnerable to our peace of mind being taken away. When the Dalai Lama was asked how he can be compassionate to the Chinese after they confiscated Tibetan land, destroyed their culture, and maimed and killed so many of his people, he answered: "They've taken everything but my [peace of] mind. I can't let them take that too." Similarly, recognizing this, a few prisoners were able to survive concentration camps as whole human beings. They bear witness to the fact that even in the most despicable circumstances imaginable, freedom is still possible (if *exceedingly* difficult). Studies on both rats and people confirm that how we react to difficulties makes an enormous difference to how we process stress. As Dr. Robert Ornstein and Dr. David Sobel concluded in their book *The Healing Brain*, it's not stress itself that causes disease, but one's reaction to stressful events.

Of course, few of us could peacefully endure the trials of Holocaust victims or the Dalai Lama, but as we move in that direction we can find a "space" and openness at times that once would have made us brittle and tense. There may even be moments when our usual annoyances strike us as amusing. Sometimes, it can seem almost silly that a little discomfort could color our whole world black. How fragile is our happiness if it relies on pleasant sensations or gets punctured by some unpleasant ones? Observing these feelings equanimously, it's clear that they change so quickly that they don't really have the power to harm or satisfy us—unless we grant them that power.

Resisting (or grabbing at) sensations creates a sense of self and tension. Try this quick exercise while either lying down or sitting: tense your whole body and then notice how the chair, bed, or sofa under you feels. You get a very clear sense of a boundary between you and the furniture. Now, try relaxing. Just melt; totally softening into whatever is holding you. Now, the line between where you end and the furniture begins isn't so clear. This shows just how much our experience can vary, depending upon our reaction and level of acceptance—and it suggests an overall direction to take.

Jesus told us that heaven is within. Our distance from that heaven, at this very moment, at all times, is our exact distance from fully accepting things just as they are.

CHAPTER 7

AWARENESS

Vipassana uses no imagination. You could imagine a sensation and that the sensation is changing even without experiencing it, but that is not reality as it is, where it is.
—*S.N. Goenka*

Whether you call it awareness, mindfulness, or just paying attention, the ability to stay focused on what is happening in the moment is generally understood as the heart of Buddhist meditation. Sometimes this is illustrated with the vignette of a young monk who asks a wizened old meditation master, "How can I become enlightened?"

"Attention," answers the ancient sage.

Unsure what to make of this, the monk asks him to elaborate. "Attention. Attention," says the teacher. Still unsatisfied, the student begs for more details. "Attention. Attention. Attention," replies the master. Hearing this, the monk bows and exits stage right.

The gist of the guru's answer is right on: if we want insight and peace of mind, it's not enough to be casually aware. We should try to be aware of everything we feel, regardless of what it is; nothing should be considered too familiar or ordinary or painful for even-handed observation. To see things as they really are and to change our unhealthy habits of mind is a full-time, moment-to-moment job. We have to keep at it and keep at it, until there are not just instants of clear awareness, but only awareness itself.

Still, one wishes the teacher hadn't been quite so laconic. What should we be aware of, and how? After all, aren't we in some sense already paying attention to whatever we experience? And even if we're half asleep, then shouldn't we be flooded with spiritual insight whenever we do concentrate really hard? Since that doesn't happen, there must be something keeping us from being fully aware. So perhaps it's wisest to consider what we are *not* aware of?

The most glaring answer is our unconscious feelings and motivations. If our goal is to be content with things as they are, and we can't do that, there must be something beyond our ordinary conscious control stopping us. We can observe this happening at any given moment. Pay close attention and try to be fully accepting of whatever is happening right now and we find, despite our best efforts, some part of us rebels.

Of course, when we're not fully aware of what we're feeling, we have no chance of becoming genuinely accepting. We fall into our old habit pattern of unconsciously reacting and categorizing our experiences on a pleasure-pain continuum. Usually we're so embroiled in fantasies, desires, or defenses we don't even notice this. But as it happens, again and again, we create patterns that, as the nun Ayya Khema observed, were never deliberately chosen, yet which direct our life, like ruts on a muddy road formed by traffic. As we continue with our blind reactions, the ruts get deeper and deeper, restricting our freedom and making it more likely we'll get stuck.

A psychotherapist friend once said, "Our overall psychological difficulties are roughly equivalent to the suffering that we're either unwilling or unable to consciously face." A healthy person has access to his dark side without being overwhelmed by it; he is not afraid to face vulnerabilities and is quick to admit mistakes. The opposite tends to be true for the troubled soul.

Since sensations are the currency of our unconscious processing, this is the place to focus. By putting our awareness there, we can start to undo our harmful impulses and begin to relieve our mind/body of tension. But just knowing this isn't enough.

Ⓒ

MENTAL CULTURE

Meditation is often understood to be a kind of concentration. In some sense that's true, concentration is needed to meditate; we need strength of mind to keep from being distracted and overwhelmed by our feelings. Yet concentration can be directed to anything. A boxer, for example, could be totally focused and aware of his body and his opponent's slightest movements, but still filled with violence. Or a camper awakened from sleep by a snapping twig could be highly sensitive to noise and motion, but gripped with fear.

It's good to remember that the Buddha taught a web of interconnected truths intended to counteract greed, hatred, and confusion. The word the Buddha used for meditation, *bhavana* means "mental development" or "mental culture." This indicates that there are qualities of mind he wanted us to develop along with awareness. Ideally our awareness should be directed toward learning how to be content, generating good will, and truthfulness. While we can't always be totally focused on our sensations (say, when we're talking to a business client), at least we can always be leaning toward one of these positive intentions.

When we sit down to meditate, our focus is on accepting and observing reality as it is. In order to experience the ultimate truth and peacefulness of nirvana, the Buddha knew we must first be aware of—to *know*, not just intellectually understand—the truths of pervasive dissatisfaction, impermanence, and selflessness (explained in detail in chapter 11). It's not a matter of consciously reminding ourselves of these, but recognizing these truths when we're seeing clearly. So our task is to keep our "vision" as clear and unbiased as possible.

As already noted, usually our awareness is so desensitized by our thoughts that we believe we're experiencing reality directly when actually we're just interpreting it. This is why equanimity is so crucial to a meditation practice: it helps keep us from falling whole hog for our agendas, expectations, and fears. At its core, meditation is devoted to cultivating awareness and equanimity in equal parts. Awareness and equanimity are like the rudder and ballast which must always be aligned and in balance to keep our insight accurate and our practice on target.

While the mind and body can never truly be separated, one can understand awareness as engaging the mind, and equanimity the body in our effort to find wisdom and peacefulness. If either of the two is missing, we drift away from wisdom. If, for example, you tried to be equanimous without being aware, you're likely to be somewhat oblivious—your serenity and tenderness lacking depth. You can keep telling yourself, "I love everybody and everything's cool," but if you're not conscious and accepting of whatever you're actually feeling at the time, you're missing unconscious desires and irritations and are as likely as ever to bonk someone when they irritate you. By paying attention to the literal sensations we experi-

ence—whether while meditating, gardening, or commuting—
we can stay grounded in a genuine equanimity. It seems to be
truly transcendent, one must be truly in touch.

MINDFULNESS MISUNDERSTOOD

The Buddha's insights into what brings happiness and our
culture's prevailing notions of the good life are so different
that it's not surprising that many misunderstand what the
Buddha meant by mindfulness. We can see this misinterpreta-
tion most clearly in the way "zen" is sometimes used as an
adjective. For example, after finishing a good run on the ski
slopes, you might overhear someone say, "I was really zen out
there." Or, in the way Zen or Buddhism is sometimes portrayed as a lifestyle—most noticeably when products are mar-
keted with taglines such as "to experience Zen living."

My intention isn't to tweak New Age advertisers or be
prudish about using the Buddha's image, and certainly not to
blame Zen, which isn't responsible for this popular adaptation. Rather, the point is to highlight how we misconstrue
what it means to "be zen" by mistaking the *ultimate* goal of
Buddhism to be to achieve a sensitive awareness. Many seem
to believe the Buddha mainly taught how to be appreciative,
centered, live simply, and be self-nurturing. These qualities are
by-products of wisdom, but they aren't the heart of it. If we
take these by-products to be the purpose of the Buddha's
path, then Buddhism turns into a stripped down hedonism—
the kind of philosophy a politically correct Hemingway would
espouse: instead of shooting lions and savoring gin, we should
try to live with gusto by treasuring every step of a forest walk
or sipping our tea as though each taste were to be our last.

Naturally, such appreciation is wonderful and it can develop along with insight, but it is definitely not the goal of the practice. If we assume the point of Buddhism is learning how to appreciate life's lovely moments or nourish our soul, we're mistaking it for another way to maximize our pleasure, as though with the right attitude our life would always feel soothing.

The Buddha intended mindfulness to be an instrument of truth and developing peace of mind, not just a method for more zestful living. It's not surprising that many of us would miss this given the prevalent currents of materialism, sensualism, and our culture's belief in the soul. Even if we don't consciously abide by these outlooks ourselves, we've absorbed some of their sentiments by osmosis. In both a superficial and deep way, the idea that we should get *something* for our efforts (as if a marvelous cup of tea is our payback for all those hours on the meditating cushion) and have soulful experiences is going to appeal to us.

The Buddha saw (and suggested we learn too) that everything is fleeting. Each moment is like a rainbow or a wave—temporary and ungraspable. So trying to savor or maintain any one of those moments, like trying to grab a wave, can only bring frustration. Once we get that, we understand the importance of not becoming attached to any experience. Then paying attention becomes an important tool not to appreciate the glow of our wood stove or the smell of spring, but to see if we're grasping for those lovely experiences. If we understand this, we're ready to begin meditating.

CHAPTER 8

HOW TO DO IT:
MEDITATION INSTRUCTIONS

We're born with this incredible instrument called a mind,
which can tune in heaven and hell and everything in between,
but no one ever gives us operating instructions on how to use
it or what to do with it. Meditation provides a way of actively
seeing into the nature and activity of this mind.
　—*John Welwood,*
　Toward a Psychology of Awakening

Thoughts and theories can be interesting, enjoyable, even life-altering. But, as we've observed, concepts can only point toward reality. Ideas tend to distort the truth, if only subtly. True wisdom comes from an understanding free of concepts.

Meditation provides a laboratory to investigate what is reality, to witness how our mind works and to learn how to become truly content. It helps us shed delusions by waking us up to this very moment. And it can show us that our life isn't as solid as we thought it was. Like the proverbial fish that doesn't notice water, we don't fully recognize what it means to be alive.

From a practical vantage point, a meditation laboratory offers a place to change the usual habit patterns of our mind without the added distractions of deadlines, agendas, and others' needs. Even those with little interest in spiritual matters usually see the benefit of spending some time every day without chasing after things, without grabbing, without reacting.

Meditation teaches us how to just be with whatever comes up. To an extent, we can all do this sometimes. Maybe your car breaks down at a busy intersection while you're running late for an appointment, and yet you're genuinely not upset. Or perhaps you unexpectedly lose your job and you remain calm, without knowing what is next. If we want to develop that capacity further—that ability to be peaceful, no matter what the circumstance—we need to practice, practice, practice. A meditation session provides the ideal training for developing that equanimity because we can focus on acceptance in isolation, recognizing clearly that any feelings or distractions that arise are coming from within us. Working in this way, even if we never find dramatic, show-and-tell spiritual insights, we're still preparing ourselves for harder, more stressful situations. So if we feel anger engulfing us, we can simply observe it—if not peacefully, then at least objectively enough so that we don't lash out.

Most people find the idea of meditating, the notion of learning how to "just be," very appealing. Intuitively we respond to it as a thirsty person does the sound of a distant stream. But we tend to project a romanticized image of what that means. Often magazines articles on meditation are accompanied by photos of people meditating in a lovely garden or meadow, the sun is shining and a few soft, billowy clouds dot the sky. You can almost hear the faint sitar music wafting in the background. Reality is considerably different. For most of us, just being often means wading through messy stuff.

As the first part of the word "*labor*atory" implies, meditation can feel like work. When we stop reacting, our accumulated tensions and desires surface. Though we feel better if we just let this discomfort pass, don't expect light and airy relaxation sessions. Meditation means facing who and what we are and that often requires us to feel things we're trying to avoid. So if you become aware of difficult or painful feelings, don't fret; odds are you're doing something right. As one vipassana teacher put it, a splinter that hurts going in will hurt coming out.

This doesn't suggest that meditating won't also feel enchanting or refreshing at times. It can be a great relief to have nothing to do but simply pay attention to this moment. And, as our life becomes purer, sitting still does become easier. Sometimes, when we least expect it, we can experience the famed "effortless effort" and a clarity and peacefulness beyond words. Yet, since we're trying to undo our tendency to reach for more, even those wonderful moments often require an effort of sorts (otherwise, we tend to try to hold on to them). Not surprisingly, most meditation sessions have both pleasant and unpleasant moments.

I hope an emphasis on effort doesn't scare off newcomers, but if you aren't prepared for some hard work, you're unlikely to stick with it or get much out of it. I've seen books on Buddhist meditation that say the meditating exercises they suggest are provocative, easy, and fun to do. Hmm. Provocative, yes, much of the time. Fun, I suppose, sometimes. But if you're expecting easy and fun, you're apt to stop when it feels boring or painful. I've met people who quit meditating because they found sitting still was difficult and decided that they "must not be cut out for it." But the truth is, it's hard for everyone—especially at first. Exercise is too, but most people understand that getting benefits from exercise requires commitment and sweat. Knowing that, they're less likely to quit when they start perspiring.

ATTITUDE

Understanding that constant change is a fact of life and that there is nothing to hold on to, we try to develop two qualities while meditating: awareness and equanimity. As S.N. Goenka says, if either of these two is weak or lacking, you will be like a bird with an injured wing or a cart with a missing wheel: you'll end up going in circles. Both awareness and equanimity are necessary for genuine tranquility and insight.

While equanimity and awareness don't exactly come naturally, as noted earlier, the two do compliment and reinforce each other. The more accepting you are, the easier it is to feel sensations, since you'll be less likely to resist what are usually considered unwanted feelings. The more aware you are, the easier it is to notice if you're frustrated or grabbing after whatever you're feeling. Still, maintaining both qualities requires some skill. If, for example, we're really *determined* to have good concentration, we may stiffen up. The best way I've found to maintain both at once is to have my body be as relaxed as possible, while also remaining alert (to do this, it helps to have the proper posture—see below for more on posture).

Though meditating can be hard work, it's not necessary to work hard. A very slight tension is needed in order to stay focused, but mainly we're opening ourselves up, not steeling ourselves against pain or pushing for a personality makeover. When painful feelings arise, if you don't struggle against them, they just don't hurt in the usual way—and the pain always, if not on our timetable, passes. And, over time, as our frustrations, self-inflicted pain, and attempts at self-protection are exposed, they dissipate at least somewhat, leaving us lighter and more energetic, since less of our energy needs to be wasted on tension.

To keep our balance, it can be helpful to remember our basic tendencies. So if you tend to push hard in life, focus a wee bit more on staying "soft"; if you're inclined to be lackadaisical, sitting up straight and concentrating on concentrating should get slightly more emphasis (in either case, don't overcompensate of course). What's important to remember is that meditation is an art. You can't set yourself on automatic pilot; each moment requires attention and balance.

It's also good to note that while persistent practice tends to develop the same positive qualities in everyone, at any given time our experience can and will vary significantly not only from other people's, but from our own, session to session and even moment to moment. It's best not to have any expectations, positive or negative. As writer Annie Lamott said of expectations, "they are resentment under construction." They interfere with seeing and being with what is. Don't try to use meditation to fix something about your life. Though that may happen on its own, if we make it our goal, we're simply wishing, not doing vipassana meditation.

Try to meditate as you would engage in a good conversation: maintain a sense of openness, without judgment or anticipating what is going to be said next. As I already noted (but almost can't emphasize too much), having an agenda prevents you from observing objectively and accepting things as they are. When you first sit down to meditate, briefly check in with yourself. Don't engage in a long monologue about your state of mind; just see how you feel, literally. There's a good chance, especially if you're new to this, you'll find an uneasiness that comes from wanting to do something else or from hoping you'll get some kind of payoff from meditating. Observe what that wanting feels like without trying to change it. Just accept that this feeling or feelings is reality for you at this moment, and that's okay—this too will pass. If you're finding you're having a lot of difficulty concentrating, it can be helpful to check in this way again.

After you finish meditating, try not to view it as, "now I'm done." See if you can maintain the sense of calm acceptance you were cultivating.

If you've meditated before using a different technique than what's described below, don't deliberately mix the two methods. It's likely, however, that when your awareness flags, your old method will sometimes "take over." No worries. When you notice it, without judgment or annoyance, simply go back to the way you were working before your old technique slipped in. That advice applies to all wanderings: when you find you've drifted, bring your awareness back to where it "should be" without disappointment. By calmly and gently bringing yourself back to your efforts, you're developing your capacity to forgive without judgment. You're also cultivating humility. Being upset with yourself for making a mistake—and this goes for any lapse—implies that someone of *my* talents shouldn't mess up. Naturally this doesn't mean we shouldn't try to do our best, but rather we shouldn't be thrown off or surprised when we fall short. Last, and most important, by inwardly smiling and calmly picking up where we were, we strengthen our efforts to be equanimous.

In some ways, meditating is like setting out on the ocean on a cold day in a very tippy kayak. To remain content or balanced (and dry), we need to be aware and accepting of our feelings. (Otherwise, our contentment isn't genuine.) That sounds easy enough, but our feelings are exactly what throw us off balance: they are either like choppy waves which tend to make us cringe and lean too far back or they're so lovely we imagine we see beautiful islands and overreach as we race ahead. In either case, we've lost our balance and are dropped in the drink. After finding ourselves all wet and cold, we tend to berate ourselves and flail about, but that only keeps us miserable longer. To get back into the boat, into the calm state we're after, requires staying relaxed and accepting—even of losing our equilibrium.

PRACTICAL STUFF

Time Commitment

Any time, even a few moments, spent meditating or improving your awareness and genuine calm is a good thing and it can't be measured in a linear way. Yet, if you really want noticeable results, try to meditate every day. At the end of a retreat, Mr. Goenka recommends the following as a minimum for daily maintenance: meditate for an hour in the morning and an hour in the evening; meditate for five minutes while lying in bed before you fall asleep and after you wake up (some may find, as I do, that those five minutes in the morning aren't all that productive as I tend to fall back asleep); meditate during "down" time—say, while waiting on line or sitting in traffic; try sitting with other vipassana meditators for one hour a week, and do at least one 10-day retreat a year.

If this still sounds like too much—and no doubt it will intimidate anyone new to this—then as the Buddhist nun and teacher Pema Chödrön says, start where you are. But before deciding you can only devote ten or thirty minutes a day, think about your priorities.

Since neither of us would enjoy a sermon about priorities, I'll just mention a few things: First, it's good to remember that if we're planning to meditate "someday," that day rarely ever comes. Second, if you really consider it important, all but the most time-downtrodden can squeeze in at least one solid block of meditation time each day. As the Dalai Lama has pointed out, he has lots of important demands on his time and he still manages to do more than four hours of spiritual exercises a day. Last, as your meditation practice develops, it's likely to give you more clarity, calm, and energy, allowing you be more efficient in your work and engaged in family life.

If you can't swing two hours a day, there's not a definitive answer to how much time you should spend meditating except the more the better. An hour block allows you to go deeper than shorter periods, but meditating twice a day is very helpful too. If forty-five minutes is the max you can spare right now, do it all in one sitting (unless your schedule only allows two twenty-plus minute sessions) and see if you can do just a few minutes in the evening (or, vice versa, if you don't have the time in the morning). If you're on a once-a-day plan, mornings are usually the best time; partly because it tends to be easier to make extra time then, but also because it sets the tone for your whole day. Note that it's generally better to meditate before meals, as after a meal you're more likely to become sleepy.

No matter what meditation schedule you settle on, try committing to it. Of course, sometimes, despite your best intentions, a day will go by without a chance to meditate. If that happens, before turning in for the night see if you can do at least a few minutes, even sitting upright in bed. That will not only keep your commitment alive in some minimum way, but give you a chance to decompress after a busy day. Even a few minutes at the end of the day can help you sleep a bit more peacefully.

Positioning Yourself

It's nice to have a regular, quiet spot set aside for meditating. It doesn't need to be anything fancy, a corner of a room will do. Meditating in the same spot creates a good atmosphere for sitting. It may sound New Agey, but by meditating in the same place, you create a kind of positive energy in that place that can be conducive to good concentration. While this positive feeling may be too subtle to notice in your home, it can be palpably felt at a meditation center. Even if you've just come from a busy day at work, it's easier to concentrate at a retreat center.

If you don't have the luxury of setting up a special sitting place, however, don't sweat it; any quiet spot will do. And if you can't find that, you may need to be resourceful. Since my house has thin walls and floors, I picked up a pair of industrial-strength headphones like those that loggers and machinists use (available from the local hardware store). They're comfortable and muffle sounds so well that I can even meditate while my daughters play loud music. With such ear protection, you could probably meditate happily under the L.A. freeway, but until you're well established in your meditation practice, it's best to meditate indoors (or at least out of the elements). Since you're trying to develop your sensitivity to sensations arising from your mindbody, even a subtle breeze can be distracting.

Once you find a spot, there's the matter of arranging yourself. If you wear a watch or glasses, remove them. Beyond that, there are some guidelines but few specifics about how you should sit and what you should do with your body parts—except your eyes and mouth. Gently close these while meditating. Closing the mouth encourages breathing through the nose. Closed eyes make it easier to turn inward. Outside stimulation distracts us from our internal life.

Sitting positions and hand placement are pretty much optional. That is, one can become just as enlightened sitting in a hard chair with your hands in your lap as you can in full lotus with thumbs delicately touching. The basic guideline is to choose a position that allows you to be relaxed yet alert, comfortable, but not cozy. Lying down tends to violate the second part of that advice. The likelihood of snoozing increases exponentially as your noggin goes south of 90° (in either direction).

The guidelines of "upright and comfortable" leave plenty of position possibilities, although there are really only three basic choices with variations: sitting on a chair, kneeling (with or without a bench or cushion), or sitting cross-legged on a cushion on a mat on the floor (half-lotus, full-lotus, or Burmese-style with legs flat). The main advantage to sitting on a cushion on the floor is that it allows for a bit more stability. Since your pelvis naturally tips forward a little in this position, you can deeply relax your body, while keeping your back straight. In the long run, this stability makes sitting on the floor the most comfortable position of all. I write "in the long run" because until you get used to it, most find sitting for long stretches on a meditation cushion can be painful.

Whichever position you choose—and feel free to try them all—it's best to stick with one for the whole length of a meditation period. A quiet body contributes to a quiet mind. Try not to move when an itch, ache, or pain appears. If your pain or itch becomes powerful, just observe the sensations that accompany it without doing anything about it. If the distraction becomes unbearable (and that's unlikely to happen if you truly just watch the sensations without wishing for them to go away), then do what you have to, but do so with awareness. It's important to see that discomfort is temporary and ever-changing, and that you don't own pain or pleasure.

No matter how you sit, it's best if your back is straight, without being tense or rigid. In *The Posture of Meditation*, body worker and long-time meditator Will Johnson notes that, as we discovered when playing with blocks as a kid, when pieces are stacked directly on top of each other, the structure is more stable. Since gravity pulls down vertically and uniformly on everything in its path, whatever doesn't have support directly below it receives uneven pressure. Applying that principle to our own spine (which has a ten pound weight on top of it), we see the importance of being aligned. Though it may take some effort at first, over time it requires less work and we can surrender without tension or collapse.

So your head should rest comfortably and evenly above your neck and spine. And your pelvis should directly support the weight of your upper body. Again, this works best if your pelvis is tipped slightly forward. Your pelvis region is then supported in turn by your meditating cushion or chair. The reason for using a meditation cushion instead of sitting directly on the floor is that without the cushion, your knees would be higher than your pelvis. In that position, the pelvis and lumbar spine tend to shift backward causing the upper torso to fold in when you relax.

We're so used to how we hold our body, we often fail to notice the tension there. Aim to have your body reflect a sense of balance, ease, and acceptance. Our body isn't just a tool that happens to be attached to our mind, but an expression of it. If our body is tense, our mind will be too. The way we settle into our meditating posture is the way we settle into meditating. If we slump, we're likely to drift into fantasy; sit ramrod straight and we're trying too hard to feel peaceful. Conversely, start daydreaming and your posture is likely to curve. Other times you may notice how when you're angry your hands actually curl into fists.

While it's a good idea to occasionally check your posture, don't obsess about it. "Am I doing it right? Are all my vertebra in line?" That kind of thinking tends to be distracting. The best time to check your posture is when you first start and if your attention has drifted for a while. As Will Johnson put it, "If the conditions of alignment and relaxation are not brought into the posture of meditation, the process of purification will still occur, but it will do so . . . more slowly."

A Do-It-Yourself Plan

There are two basic steps to learning vipassana. Step one is called ānāpāna or working with the breath; the second part, traditionally known as vipassanā-bhāvanā, works with sensations throughout the body. Vipassana is taught on day four of a 10-day retreat.

Within these two basic steps, there are also smaller steps. Learning the whole meditation technique is a gradual process. During a course, roughly every day and a half you change or add a new focus, which is usually only subtly different from the previous one. Each new aspect of the technique builds upon what you've already learned, helping you develop greater concentration and awareness. Each new focus requires a more subtle attention than the one before it, which sharpens the mind. All together, there are seven stages or parts to learning this technique.

During a retreat one formally meditates for ten to eleven hours a day. So it takes more than 100 hours of intensive meditation to be introduced to the technique—or fourteen-plus hours per stage. Since one's concentration and effort is likely to be much stronger at a course than at home, I recommend *at least* doubling that time. In other words, shoot for spending a minimum of roughly thirty hours meditating with each aspect of the technique when learning it on your own. So if you meditate for two hours a day, each stage would take about two weeks to complete, or three and a half months for absorbing the whole technique. If you only meditate half an hour a day, each stage would take two months— or a bit over a year to learn the entire thing.

This timeline is only a rough guideline. What's more important is seeing if you can consistently concentrate well, for at least short periods of time before moving on to the next phase. So for the ānāpāna stages, if you've put in your thirty hours per, but you can't maintain a strong focus for *at least* a minute at a time, continue working with that aspect of the technique until you can. Likewise, for the vipassanā-bhāvanā stages, except here the minimum should be at least three minutes of good concentration, but preferably five. Of course, don't actually time yourself; these are just approximate guidelines to give you a sense of what you need to work on.

Even if you've practiced other meditating techniques for years, it's best to start at the beginning. This doesn't suggest you haven't benefited from other forms of meditation; clearly your concentration is likely to be better than someone who's never meditated before, but to give this technique a fair trial, it's best to start fresh. Keep in mind that even the most experienced meditators, including S.N. Goenka, begin every retreat with ānāpāna.

Though each stage of learning the method builds on the one before it, I purposely avoided identifying them with a letter or number because I didn't want to imply a ranking or hint that you should be anxious to move ahead. Try not to rush through any part of the technique, just as you would try to appreciate a whole mountain's trail without just scurrying to the top. By scrambling for a prize, not only will we miss the subtleties on the journey, we're likely to be somewhat disappointed with the view since we exaggerate what the reward will be. Each step has its own texture, interest, difficulties, rewards, and purpose. Focusing on breathing can bring powerful and subtle concentration. The Buddha is said to have reached very deep states of concentration while working with his breath—training that was necessary for him to have the strength and openness of mind to become enlightened.

Even vipassana meditators who have done countless courses may, at times, return to their breath, not only at the beginning of a retreat, but if they're having difficulty concentrating. Likewise, you may need to return to the "beginning" techniques at any point when you're having trouble focusing. Sometimes meditating can bring up very powerful feelings. In fact, the very effectiveness of the technique may release long-held emotions. Often this happens after we've been meditating "well," when you feel you've been making progress. These strong emotions can be like large waves: if we're not prepared for them they seem to crash down on us. When we face the wave directly, though, diving straight into it, we realize it's just water and we can manage. Still, sometimes the best we can do is batten down the hatches. That's when focusing on breathing can be very helpful. Another alternative when you're feeling overwhelmed (assuming you've already been working with your body sensations) is to focus on the feelings in your arms and legs (these parts generally don't hold our most powerful feelings, which tend to accumulate in our stomach, chest, back, and neck).

As you read through the instructions below, don't sweat the details at first. In fact, *initially*, it's a good idea to read quickly through "The Instructions" section of this chapter (up to the part that describes doing Metta). This way you'll get a general sense of what the technique entails and still have a fresh, beginner's mind when you're actually ready to meditate. Once you are meditating according to a particular set of instructions, then it's best to read that section severals times—not at one sitting, but at various times before you meditate. Simple as the instructions seem, it's still helpful to hear them many times. During a retreat, the same basic instructions are repeated again and again. Yet even if you've heard them hundreds of times, the repetition is still helpful. We all have a strong proclivity to hear what we want to hear, making it easy to misconstrue even simple directions. We tend to forget things that our wiser half already knows. Changing old habits requires consistent re-minders.

Also, before sitting down to meditate you might want to try reading a page or two of Buddhist teachers whose writings you find inspiring—with the caveat that if the inspiration includes directions for a different meditation method, ignore that part.

Last, at the end of each meditation session, take at least a few minutes to practice Metta (described in detail below). Metta is a way of developing loving-kindness and sharing your meditation practice with others.

THE INSTRUCTIONS

ĀNĀPĀNA

The Touch of the Breath

This meditation is very simple. Breathing naturally, observe the sensations the touch of the breath makes in the area of the nostrils—inside the nostrils, at their entrance, or just below the nostrils. It doesn't matter which of these small nasal spots you focus on, or if you're aware of all these small spots at once. The important thing is to be concentrating on the feeling the breath causes in a small area, both with the in and out breath. Although you're working with the breath, don't concentrate on the breath itself, only on the sensations it creates.

Don't try to control your breathing. Don't imagine or visualize the breath or think about it. And drop any notions you may have about breathing. Don't, for example, as some methods recommend, picture your breath going into your lungs. Do not say to yourself "breathing in; breathing out." And don't count your breaths. All your attention should go to noticing the sensations your breath causes in your nostril area and ignoring everything else. What's most important to remember, and this applies to every aspect of this method, is that you should try to focus just on what is, not what you hope for or imagine. Essentially, you're training yourself to be with whatever is, without anything added.

While this meditation is simple, it's definitely not easy. Your thoughts are likely to wander again and again. While your goal is to be like a sentry at a gate, you're more likely to be a deserter, chasing fantasies within a short time of taking up your post. Not to worry though, that's to be expected, especially if you're new to this. (In fact, if you can do five continuous minutes without drifting you're doing really well.) Each time your attention wanders, patiently bring it back to the breathing-induced sensations in your nostril area. Don't get down on yourself for messing up, and don't celebrate sustained awareness. Strive for relaxed vigilance and tolerance. Try not to sacrifice one at the expense of the other.

Watching your breath like this, you're likely to notice the variety and subtle differences that occur. The sensations accompanying our breath are forever changing and more amorphous than we normally think. No two breaths are or feel the same. Like watching a river's current or ocean waves, these subtly changing patterns can be fascinating. But don't turn your watching into a game; keep your awareness choiceless, desireless. Accept whatever sensations arise, even those in other parts of your body, without diverting your attention from your nasal area.

There's no cause for alarm if one of your nostrils is blocked or if your breathing is very shallow. As your mind calms down, your breathing is likely to become very soft. If we observe ourselves closely, we discover that when we become agitated our breath gets stronger. Should that happen, don't try and change it. Let your breath be natural, unless you find you're consistently spacing out for more than five minutes (again, don't actually time it). If that happens, try taking a few deliberate, slightly hard breaths to refocus your attention. But after a few hard breaths, go back to breathing naturally. Also, if you must shift positions, take some deliberate breaths while moving, as it will help you maintain your concentration. As much as possible, you want to be continuously aware of feeling your breath in your nostril area. As Mr. Goenka says, "continuity is the secret of success." This also applies to times when you're not officially meditating. See if you can have some awareness of the feeling of the breath in the nostrils area when you're driving, taking a walk, or relaxing on the sofa.

The Mustache

With a calm and attentive mind, keep your attention in the triangular area below the nostrils and above your upper lip. Observe *any* sensations that occur in this limited area, not just those feelings caused by breathing. Don't look for any particular type of sensation; just notice what is there. You may feel itchy, you may feel trembling, you may feel warmth, cold, perspiration, breeze, pain, palpitation, jiggling, wiggling, pulsating or any combination of these. It can be any sensation at all. It doesn't matter. The important thing is to simply feel sensations without trying to make them go away or change them (that happens on its own anyhow). Whatever you notice, don't label it. Simply observe, observe, observe with total acceptance of whatever you're feeling. Note the difference between looking for something and just looking. After observing sensations equanimously, you will delve deeper and experience them in what seems like a new, interesting, even pleasant way. Before you know it, you may begin craving and looking for that more interesting view. This interferes with an investigative, open mind—a mind that observes just what is.

Attend to your small mustache area as though you were a fully engaged, yet unbiased scientist doing an experiment—which, in fact, is what you are doing. When you meditate or observe equanimously, you are a scientist of your existence, in essence working to test and reproduce results that the Buddha first discovered more than 2,500 years ago. The Buddha came to these truths by experiencing life without ideas about the way things should be. When meditating, we are trying to wake up from the barrier thoughts create. Be with what is real, not imagined or hoped for. When we see without any biases, the truth of this moment reveals itself.

If you find it consistently difficult to feel sensations, try holding your breath for half a minute and notice the sensations that creates. This can "jump start" an awareness of sensations, but if this doesn't work, feel free to switch back to focusing on the sensations breathing makes in your nostril area, as you did in the first stage. Don't consider this a setback. A sensation is a sensation; you can make good use of any and all of them. But once you're able to focus reasonably well again, come back to feeling any and all sensations in the mustache area again—either later during the same meditation session, the next day, or next week.

Fingertip

To sharpen your awareness and concentration further, restrict your focus in the area between your nostrils and upper lip to a spot the size of the tip of your finger. Again, see what you feel—without judging, without expectations, without thoughts of me, mine, I. As your awareness loses the running commentary and opens to what is actually happening in the moment, you'll notice everything is constantly changing. This ever-moving dance, this swirling and unfolding of impersonal phenomenon, leaves nothing to hold on to. Nothing to grasp. Yield to the sensations. Be defenseless. While you're likely to try to assess how you're doing and wonder if you are a "good meditator," this is a fruitless (and ironic) question. Such questions are attempts to bolster the ego and get a grip on things. But there is no handle to grab on to. Reality is a constant flow; continue to patiently and persistently experience whatever sensations unfold. Don't look for anything special. Simply look.

During an evening discourse, Goenkaji tells the story of a successful and wealthy businessman who took his first 10-day meditation course during a Burmese heat wave. This man (a friend of his) was an intelligent fellow and meditated with great determination, but he claimed he couldn't feel any sensations. Like everyone else at the course, he was told a sensation can be anything—pain, perspiration, pressure, a sense of heat, itching, throbbing, stinging, tickling, prickling, hunger, burning, tension, hardness, etc. Yet despite the repeated instructions, this guy maintained he wasn't feeling any sensations. One time, Goenkaji, visited him in his meditation cell. His friend was drenched in sweat and had rolled up his sleeves and pant legs. "Are you feeling any sensations?" Goenkaji asked. "No, still nothing," he answered as he wiped his brow. He was looking for something unusual, something mystical. He didn't take ten days out of his busy schedule to feel "ordinary" sensations.

When we hear this vignette, that businessman sounds so silly, but we're often more like him than we realize. As one practices this technique, you notice that even when we're not distracted, unconsciously we regularly "reject" sensations. What we're doing is looking for something special (usually that means pleasant) or we want to avoid an unpleasant sensation (including feeling bored). We often overlook our most familiar sensations because we're so used to them we can hardly notice them anymore. They seem to just be part of the fabric of the world, as opposed to just another sensation. The result is we're deaf to much of what we feel. On, and especially off, the meditating cushion, we ignore, edit, and filter. The less we do this, the more sensitive we'll become. A Buddha is called an "awakened one" because he or she is without filters; there are no blocks in his or her awareness. He or she is totally open.

If you find yourself unable to concentrate on this small spot, as before, hold your breath for thirty seconds or so to heighten your awareness of sensations. Also, if you need to, feel free to go back to one of the earlier techniques—try feeling all sensations in the mustache area first, and if that doesn't help, go back to experiencing the touch of the breath.

Q

VIPASSANA:
WORKING WITH YOUR BODILY SENSATIONS

Body Scan Head to Toe

The full body scan is the heart of this meditation technique. There are variations and refinements of the scan, but the instructions in this section provide the main tool for developing experiential wisdom.

Start by bringing an acute yet gentle attention to the top of your head, to the spot on your skull which indents slightly—the area that would be the "soft spot" if you were an infant. Don't picture the spot, but just try to feel whatever sensations you can in that area. Again, the sensations you feel can be anything—tingling, itching, vibrating, prickling, tickling, twitching, etc. Don't assume you know what sensations you're going to feel. Rather, it should be as if whatever sensations you're experiencing there you are feeling for the first time.

After feeling the top of your head, move on, observing the sensations throughout your scalp, then the back of your head, and your face. The aim is to bring awareness to sensations everywhere on the surface of your body. Be sure to cover your ears, behind your ears, inside your ears, the skin beneath your eyebrows, your eyelids, your nose, your lips, etc. We have a strong tendency to visualize the body part we're focusing on instead of just experiencing it. But visualizing something means you're imagining it, not just observing what is. If you notice yourself visualizing, just bring yourself back to the sensations themselves.

After you've covered your head, continue on to your neck, both front, back, and underneath the chin. From there move to your collarbone area and head down your left or right shoulder, covering everywhere on your arm, including the elbow, hand, fingers, and in-between your fingers. If you did the left arm first, then do your right next (or vice versa).

The first several times you do this mediation, go slowly and carefully, yet without stopping. You want to keep your attention moving. As soon as you feel a sensation, move on, covering roughly two to three inch sections at a time. After you've done the technique a few times, you can pick up the pace somewhat—as long as you don't gloss over sensations in any body part. In the beginning, the sequencing may feel mechanical, but over time it comes to feel natural as your awareness tends to flow over your body.

In some places it will be easy to feel sensations and in others hard. Either way, once you feel a sensation, move on. If your concentration is good you can do a thorough head to foot scan in about ten minutes. Other times in may take an hour. But the time it takes isn't important. What is important is focusing on the sensations themselves, trying to maintain a soft, investigative and equanimous mind. A mind that doesn't try to create, seek out, or reject any sensation. It's almost impossible to remind yourself of that too much, as our tendency is to not be open to everything we feel.

It's good to remember that an essential quality of all sensations is that they are ephemeral. As Mr. Goenka says at the beginning of many meditation sessions, "anicca, anicca, anicca," which is Pali for "changing, changing, changing." When we really realize that everything we experience is so fleeting, then the futility of grasping after or recoiling from any sensation becomes self-evident. So it's helpful to cultivate an awareness of how all our sensations are changing, yet without making it a deliberate thought.

Continuing on with the body scan, investigate your torso—your chest, your armpits, your sides, your stomach. Yes, without reacting or fanfare, examine your pubic and genital areas as well. After your front comes your back, your shoulders, your middle back, lower back, and bum. It doesn't matter whether you do the front or back first, but for now be consistent. Maintaining the same basic pattern allows you to develop a regular and easy flow that frees you to concentrate on sensations. It also helps insure you won't miss any spots.

If you feel a strong sensation such as a sharp pain or itching in, say, your foot while you're scanning your back, don't jump to the strong sensation; stay focused on the back without disrupting your "route." Don't try to make the pain or whatever you're feeling go away (which you wouldn't be able to do anyhow), but don't give it any importance either. Often the "unbearable" itch or pain will be gone by the time you come to it, but if it's still there, you can take a bit more time observing it.

A thorough, nonreactive investigation into a strong sensation can dissipate or deconstruct it (as long as you're not trying to banish it while you're observing it). Putting the laser of awareness on a "gross" sensation reveals that it's actually made up of fleeting, dancing, finer, more delicate and intricate sensations. This awareness can change the whole character of the feeling. Don't work to make this happen; it will happen on its own if you observe keenly and equanimously. (Did I mention it's important to be accepting and without expectations?)

Try not to stay more than a minute or so with any single sensation—or if it's a really powerful one, no more than five minutes. It's great to see that feelings which seem so "solid" really aren't substantial after all. But it's best to avoid making difficult feelings your main focus—and you don't want to jump around from one powerful feeling to another. This would hinder developing a keen and subtle awareness.

What's left to scan now is your legs on down. Investigate the thigh, the knee, the back of the knee, the calf, the ankle, the whole foot, the toes, and in-between the toes. Again, it doesn't matter which leg comes first. After you've finished with your last big or little toe, start back at the top of your head again. Should you find that you've spaced out for a while and "lost your place," go to the spot you last remember covering and continue from there.

If you come to a "blind" spot, a place where you can't feel anything, keep your attention in that area for up to a minute or so until you feel something, anything. Be patient. Sensations are certainly there, but sometimes they are too subtle or scary for us to bring awareness to them. Should the spot remain "blank," however, see if you can feel what this "nothing" feels like. Does it have any qualities or characteristics to it? As meditation teacher Wes Nisker asks, "Does this nothing feel like numbness, or more like a voidness or empty space?" If investigating the nothingness still doesn't turn up anything, try to feel the touch of cloth on that spot (if it's covered with clothing), or to detect any air currents there. Wherever there is life there is sensation, so some feeling is there. But if you still can't feel anything after a bit, don't worry or feel you're doing anything wrong. Move on, and eventually you'll feel that part either on the next round or at some other point, as long as you stick with the practice.

Toe to Head—and Back Again

Relaxed yet attentive, start at the top of your head again. Remember that while you are conducting an inquiry into your mind-body, this is not a conventional inquiry. You're not interested in finding concrete answers or solutions, but in getting insight into what it really feels like to be alive. You're opening to the mystery, even the confusion, of whatever is, of what is nameless—without trying to understand in the sense that you can wrap a concept around it.

From your head move your attention throughout your body, piece by piece, part by part, as described in the "Body Scan Head to Toe" section above. Be aware of the impermanent, forever changing nature of sensations. Sensations will come and sensations will go, regardless of our plans for them. You can't choose your sensations, but you can choose how you respond to them. Resisting, cringing, or trying to get rid of a feeling only tends to intensify it. Any of the sensations we experience while meditating are from the resurfacing of previous moments of grasping or recoiling. When our mind gets quiet, it's easier to notice that unsatisfied, frustrated energy. Reacting to these feelings only reinforces the very feelings that are making us uncomfortable in the first place. Try not to get snagged on the rebound (see chapter 11 for a more detailed explanation of how this works).

All the guidelines from the first body scan apply here too, but instead of stopping at the toes, switch directions and move awareness back up your leg. Work in reverse order up to the crown of the head again. Once there, back down you go, and so on. Remember, even though we say bring awareness to your body, your body and mind are inseparable. Full awareness of your whole body is full awareness of your whole mind. For this reason you don't want to overlook any place or neglect blind spots (except temporarily if you can't feel anything for roughly a minute).

Ideally try to keep the body scans from becoming mechanical. If you feel you're going through the motions, try changing your scanning pattern. If you've regularly been working horizontally, go vertically for a while, making stripes or working in a spiral fashion, swirling your way down and up your body. As long as you don't miss any spots, you can be playful with different patterns, keeping two caveats in mind: avoid a pattern that's so intricate it distracts you from the awareness of sensations, and don't bounce around between patterns so much that deciding on a pattern becomes a distraction.

If your mind is dull or you're having trouble feeling sensations, try bringing awareness to big chunks of your body. For example, you could experience your right thigh, your whole face, or a side of your face at once. Then, gradually try to reduce the size of the area. If this doesn't help your concentration or you're agitated, you can always go back to focusing on sensations from your breath or on the small area below the nostrils and above the upper lip. Working with the breath in this way can be alternated with focusing on the sensations in your extremities until you feel calmer.

As always, feel sensations without identifying them or with them. Again, remember acceptance, acceptance, acceptance; know that everything changes, changes, changes. Indeed, every sensation we feel indicates things are changing.

Free Flow

After you've been meditating with the body scan a while, you may spontaneously find times when thoughts disappear, sensations turn into pure energy, and your awareness becomes very subtle. Awareness flows easily either through a particular body part or through your whole body. This feels quite pleasant. You may even get the sense that you're totally disappearing.

This experience of complete dissolution is traditionally called *bhanga*. Bhanga is significant, as it reveals our lack of solidity. Once strong, gripping feelings and thoughts disappear or wane, and our minds become quiet, we experience what feels like pure awareness or that our body is comprised of very subtle arising and passing vibrations.

While this partial or total dissolution is noteworthy, it should be approached with some caution. Not because anything bad happens to you, but because it is so pleasant, even exciting. Bhanga and free flows are seductive. Soon enough we start craving the lovely energy flow. It feels good, it's kind of neat, and we take it to mean we are good meditators, spiritually advanced souls. Naturally, try not to fall for this line of thinking.

Goenkaji repeatedly warns against playing the game of sensations; that is, working to get pleasant, interesting sensations and getting frustrated or down when they disappear. As S.N. Goenka says, this is what we've been doing our whole life: chasing what feels good and ignoring or running from what doesn't. A sensation is a sensation. Although free flow is helpful to show our essential lack of substance, what you're really working on is developing a nongrasping mind.

Since you can't force free flow, there's really no point in pining for it anyhow. One of the preconditions of it "appearing" is that you're fully accepting of whatever is happening at the moment; so the very thoughts that crave the free flow prevent it from happening. Still, if you experience free flow, here's what you do: Pass your attention quickly up and down your whole body. Don't overlook any body parts, but your attention will be more diffused than a part-by-part scan. This movement up and back will feel natural as there aren't any obstructions and your concentration will be good. After going head-to-toe and toe-to-head a few times, go back to small part-by-part awareness.

Even if you aren't spontaneously experiencing free flow, in-between rounds of part-by-part checking, sometimes try one or two quick, more diffused scans. Mr. Goenka calls this quicker, larger scanning "sweeping en masse" (*en masse* is French for all together). If your awareness flows through some parts and not others, that's fine; sweep where you can and pass your attention through each individual part where you can't. Should symmetrical parts of your body—say, both your arms and/or your legs or front and back torso—have similar, subtle sensations at the same time, you may observe them together, simultaneously.

If you aren't able to free flow at all and find the quick rounds of scanning distracting, then just go back to the smaller section investigating you had been doing before. Remember, a sensation is a sensation. Awareness and equanimity can be developed on any feeling.

Everything, Everywhere

As you work your way through your mind-body with nonattached, gentle awareness, inch by inch, moment by moment, you're working your way to the truth about your existence. It can be a hard, seemingly unending effort; sometimes you'll want to crawl out of your skin. But if you continue working in the right way, be confident you are making progress, lightening your load, freeing yourself from long-held, unconscious energy that creates frustration and unhappiness.

The last piece to add to a complete, full body scan is an internal investigation. So after a round of scanning the sensations on the body's surface part by part, from head to toe and toe to head, and after a round of sweeping en masse, go inside. With penetrating, thorough awareness, go through the whole body. Starting at the head, investigate the sensations in your brain, eyeballs, tongue, and jaw. Move your awareness left to right, right to left. Front to back, back to front. Continue moving down in this thorough, noticing-everything-in-the-cross-section-of-awareness way. Check inside your neck, your arms and hands, your torso, all the way to your feet—and back.

Observe in a way that takes nothing for granted. Observe without expectations, without hopes for results. Be desireless. Although you're working to develop equanimity, don't crave it. Craving is craving. Hungering even for peacefulness heads us in the opposite direction. Be patient and let things unfold as they will.

It's easy to tell ourselves we want to be accepting, yet fully softening to all our sensations, no matter how unpleasant, is often another story. We're built to avoid pain and discomfort, so we usually distract, recoil, or numb ourselves rather than feel. This tendency is the basis of our rationalizations and our attempts to create a golden self-image. This avoidance impulse, which keeps us from fully experiencing this moment, is brought into the light when we meditate. The effort of meditating comes from consciously softening and staying with what is happening rather than skirting away. Even after lots of experience, we still resist the hard, the boring, the irritating. Looked at closely, the feeling that accompanies this resistance, could be expressed as "anything but this." As though what we're now experiencing is as hard as it gets. It's not. We can open to any sensation, difficult as it may initially seem.

Bringing your awareness inside, you can see there is no solidity anywhere. Sensations are on the surface, sensations are inside, but nothing is fixed or constant anywhere. It's all moving, changing energy. Don't label what you feel, don't resist it; just be aware. After you've systematically checked your sensations everywhere, feel free to occasionally check yourself at random. Can you feel inside a nostril? Throughout your spine? Behind your left knee?

It's important to remember that no matter what the quality of the sensation you're experiencing—whether solid and strong or subtle and flowing—it doesn't matter. Don't try to change any sensation you're having or be disappointed because you're not having the ones you want. You can work in different ways according to the type of sensations you're experiencing: free flowing with subtle sensations and going part by part with "grosser" feelings. Every sensation offers an excellent opportunity to work on acceptance. Painful or unpleasant sensations are great for working on our inclination to recoil; pleasant ones are ideal for observing without getting caught by our tendency to be greedy and grasping. Since it's actually easier to be nongrasping of difficult feelings (who wants them anyhow?), in a way one can feel grateful for them since they help us progress. As Goenkaji says, the best benchmark of "success" is the balance of your mind. Are you able to be accepting, truly accepting?

Even if we only catch glimpses of the kind of freedom and loss of boundaries that is possible through this practice, we've seen an opening. If it feels right, trust it; it can be deepened, bringing us real peace of mind.

Metta

It's good to remember that we meditate to benefit everyone, not just ourselves. In fact, we can't really be happy ourselves unless we wish others well. So after meditating, spend at least a few minutes consciously sharing your best intentions. In this tradition, practicing metta is the only time we deliberately use words while meditating.

Start by checking in with yourself and focusing attention on bodily sensations. Before doing metta, see if you have any anger or negative feelings. If you do, wait or do it another time. Since you're sending "out" your energy, you want it to be positive. Then, with a calm, strong mind, say slowly and to yourself things that express your wish for every being to do well. Things like: "May all beings be peaceful. May all beings be kind. May all beings be happy." If you prefer some other sentiments that profess good spiritual tidings and are more meaningful for you, use those. It's fine to repeat the same phrases over and over or use new ones that reflect your good intentions of that moment.

As you say these words, try to radiate your energy/sentiments out into the world, sharing them as wholeheartedly as you can. Try repeating the last word or words of the phrase you're saying a few times—creating the sense that your sentiments are echoing or generating ever-increasing ripples in a lake.

Wishing others well combined with awareness of our feelings can be a powerful spiritual tool to combat strong feelings of negativity. Say, for instance, someone insults us. With strong mindfulness, it's possible to equanimously observe the feelings that creates in us and let them pass, but for most of us, especially off the meditating cushion, that would be very hard to do without wanting to strike back or without spinning tales of revenge and injustice. By wishing the best for the insulter, we can help keep the vengeful, self-righteous thoughts and feelings we have from raging out of control. It's important to remember we're not trying to suppress our feelings (and that's why remaining mindful of our sensations can be so helpful), but hoping to avoid feeding the fires of our anger. In this way we're not squashing true feelings, just containing them so they don't lead to feelings and intentions that ultimately cause more harm.

PRACTICE-RELATED Q&A

 I felt a sharp and odd pain during the last meditation session; is this normal?

If instead of "a sharp and odd pain," you substituted a specific "ailment"—such as "a stabbing pain in my neck," "my ears started ringing," "my knee felt like it was burning"—this would be the most common question new meditators ask at a retreat.

If we remember that these uncomfortable, painful, and sometimes scary sensations are tension being released, we realize they actually offer a good opportunity. By not reacting to these powerful feelings, we can at least partially release them. While this may be easier to advise than do, it's quite possible, even liberating. Besides, taking the opposite tact—resisting, fighting, or trying to make unwanted feelings go away—doesn't really work and only reinforces the very feelings you're struggling against. If instead of opposing these hard sensations, you observe even the toughest ones with a relaxed and accepting mind, they will pass. Perhaps they won't go away immediately, but when you're truly accepting (again, that doesn't mean you're doing it *so that* what's annoying you will go away), the quality of an unpleasant feeling changes and becomes, well, acceptable.

When very painful sensations arise, some instinctive part of us contracts, afraid we're going to be grievously injured or die. As far as I know, this has never happened. If you've started meditating in a comfortable position, even if your knees are burning, you won't be doing any physical damage to yourself (unless perhaps you have an old injury that makes lotus-position type maneuvering unwise for you). In fact, since we're reducing stress, meditating, if anything, improves our health, including our flexibility.

To use a limited analogy, we can think of the difficult times we face when meditating as the equivalent of jogging up hills; not giving up really increases our health. Unlike marathon running, however, strength through endurance doesn't suggest a grin-and-bear-it attitude. Remember, it's stick-to-it-ness combined with letting go that allows us to be accepting of the hard stuff. If, despite your best efforts to calmly observe difficult sensations, you really feel overwhelmed, try concentrating on sensations from your breath. And of course when you're in pain, you can always shift positions as well, but try to do so in a conscious, non-reactive way.

Q *I get sleepy a lot when I meditate. Is there anything I can do?*

Drowsiness can definitely be a problem. Our unconscious mind can be wickedly clever at avoiding anything it doesn't like. What better avoidance technique than grogginess, since unlike sharp pain, it's very difficult to observe sleepiness without succumbing to it? This is one reason we get drowsy once when start meditating, even if we had been feeling wide awake before we sat down.

Some Buddhist traditions recommend meditating with your eyes open to help prevent falling asleep. While this may help a bit, it's not enough to outweigh the benefits that come from having your internal sense of awareness enhanced by closing your eyes. Besides, when you're sleepy, meditating with eyes open barely seems to help anyhow. Like trying to stay awake when you're driving, telling yourself to keep the lids up is generally a losing battle when they feel heavy.

There are a few things one can do to contend with drowsiness. One, as mentioned earlier, is to meditate on an empty stomach. The blood used to digest our food increases the likelihood of drowsiness. Another is to keep a light on if it's dark out. Even with our eyes closed, light affects us in a wakeful way. You can also try picking up the pace of your scanning. This adds a touch of liveliness to our awareness. If none of these help, try meditating standing up for five minutes or so and then sitting back down again. You may even need to do this several times. Should that fail, there's always splashing a bit of water on your face and/or going for a short walk before another attempt.

If your sleepiness seems to be beyond avoidance and into sheer fatigue, there may be little you can do at that moment outside of taking the nap you need, and then trying again later. Sometimes when we're really busy and crunched, fatigue overcomes us when we slow down. If this is happening to you a lot, fixing the problem may require a whole life adjustment.

Q *Why not just let sensations unfold and notice whatever arises?*

If we only observed those feelings that call out the loudest, we wouldn't develop the keen awareness necessary to notice subtler sensations. Some of our conditioning and attachments are very subtle. It can be difficult for us to notice the ways in which we manipulate or are manipulated by certain feelings. Honing our sensitivity makes us more likely to be conscious, regardless of the feeling or circumstance. Much of our life is missed because we dismiss what we're doing as mundane.

When not meditating, try to be aware of any sensation you feel. This gives us plenty of "free-form" time.

Q Is it helpful to identify the emotional content of the sensations we experience?

Sometimes you'll spontaneously become aware of an emotional event associated with sensations. When passing my attention across my cheek during my first retreat, for example, I felt a stinging at the same time I had a memory of my brother slapping me across the face. This had happened when I was a kid and I hadn't thought of it in years, but obviously in some way it was still there. Most of the time, however, there isn't such a clear connection between a sensation and an emotional memory. More often such associations are manifest in thought snippets or tangential thoughts that may set us off into reveries after experiencing certain sensations (although we usually don't recognize this).

If emotional insights—either through clear connections or thought snippets—happen spontaneously, so much to the good. This awareness can help us understand ourselves better, but don't make such psychological insight the purpose of your meditation. Psychotherapy is better suited for this work.

Meditation is for purifying one's mind. Psychological insights may well come from meditating, but it's a byproduct— it's the molasses you get when making sugar. Likewise, meditation can improve your physical health, but meditating with this in mind makes it less likely to happen. When you have an agenda, you start to want and crave and you lose the objectivity and equanimity which helps us heal naturally.

Last, trying to gather psychological insight from individual sensations while meditating is distracting. As Mr. Goenka said, "It would be as if someone washing a dirty cloth stopped to check what caused each stain on the cloth. This wouldn't help him do his job, which is only to clean the cloth."

Q   *I sometimes have exciting brainstorms while meditating; is there any harm in taking a quick break from meditating and jotting them down?*

Since meditating tends to give us clarity of thought while also releasing us from the pressures that inhibit creativity, it's not uncommon to have insightful thoughts while we're sitting there. There are several reasons to resist jotting down these brilliant gems, though. The main one is that meditation is designed for developing purity of heart and mind. If we bring in other motives, we're sure to fall short of this mark.

For a meditation practice to be effective, we must be really committed to it, not only over time, but also while actually doing it. If we think of the time we set aside for meditating as also time to pursue our creative or artistic interests, we won't have the concentration or equanimity necessary to meditate well, ironically killing or crippling the "golden goose" which was leading to insights in the first place.

It's also good to remember that thoughts which mesmerize us are often unconscious distractions designed to combat uneasiness. Thinking of a money-making business idea, for example, can help comfort our worries about losing our job; figuring out the plot for the next great American screenplay lets us imagine ourselves as an artistic savant, covering over feelings of inadequacy. I often find that ideas that seemed so clever while I was meditating turn out to be considerably less dazzling—or even a bit dopey—after considering them more carefully.

If, despite knowing all this, you have some smashing idea that's important to you and you're so concerned you'll forget it later that it becomes a big distraction, then (assuming you're meditating alone) simply and mindfully adjust something that's by your cushion in a odd way—say put your watch in your shoe or turn your alarm clock upside down—and then let go of the idea. You'll be sure to remember your idea when the oddly placed object jogs your memory.

Q *I'm trying my best to concentrate, but still space out a lot. Is there anything I can do?*

Some drifting simply comes with the territory. Unless, you're a very advanced meditator or have been at a retreat for several days, everyone spends a bit of time lost in fantasy. As with any skill we try to hone, the main thing to do is try, try again without getting disappointed. Keep in mind that an awareness practice is a job for a scientist, not a judge; so don't issue any verdicts. Mindfulness itself shouldn't feel onerous, but, if anything, freeing. Remember, it is always now, which is the only time we can ever be aware of.

Often when we're trying hard but not concentrating well, it's because we're looking for something. Maybe we had a great meditation session yesterday and want to feel like that again, or maybe we read something inspiring so we end up wanting to experience something extraordinary. While effort is usually necessary to concentrate well, sometimes we can try too hard. If you notice yourself doing this (or even if you don't notice it but find you're not concentrating well), check how relaxed and accepting you are. To be truly mindful we also need to be equanimous.

An often-overlooked aspect of concentrating well is that we forget to consider the problem in the context of our whole life. If our life is frantic or filled with conflict, then how can we expect to sit down and be calm like a Buddha? The way one really starts making progress on this path is by recognizing that everything we do and even think affects us in many ways. Being kind, directly addressing and trying to resolve frictions in our life, and maintaining the precepts (see chapter 12) all help make us more centered on the meditation cushion.

CHAPTER 9

IS THIS REALLY HOW THE BUDDHA
WANTED US TO MEDITATE?

There may be different techniques. We don't say that this is the only way. But what I am teaching is universal. Anybody can practice it, from any religion or tradition, and they will get the same result. We have people coming to vipassana courses from every religion in the world. I don't tell them, "Convert yourself from this religion to that religion." My teacher never asked me to convert to a religion. The only conversion is from misery to happiness.
    —S.N. Goenka

At times, it seems as if everyone wants a piece of the Buddha. Sometimes in a figurative, even playful way, as with the book titled *If the Buddha Dated.* Or sometimes literally: there was a sect in Ceylon, for instance, which revered Gautama's left eye tooth for eleven hundred years. The Buddha's authority and stamp of approval carries a lot of weight.

Nearly every branch of Buddhism claims direct lineage to the man himself. As unlikely as this initially sounds (and some scholars are skeptical), it's at least theoretically possible. The Buddha trained many monks. Those disciples then trained others who trained others; each teacher, influenced by his own insights and ideas, may have changed the emphasis slightly. So it's natural that over time the seeds of the Buddha's wisdom—planted in the soil of different cultures and pruned according to the style of its caretakers—would grow into a lush forest with diverse foliage.

During the fifty-five years the Buddha taught, he gave tens of thousands of discourses, adjusting his teaching and emphasis according to whom he was speaking to. He used many metaphors and methods to make his points. This varied approach can lead one to conclude that there are many paths to enlightenment. And it's a conclusion that's hard to argue with, since there seem to be enlightened beings in all traditions, Buddhist and otherwise.

True sages in various traditions may share many common traits and insights, implying there may even be underlying, if not fully recognized, similarities in how they arrived at their wisdom. But even if we found common links, the diversity of wise folks and traditions inspires humility about taking one's own way as *the* way; it highlights the importance of holding any claims to orthodoxy gently.

The Buddha often emphasized the importance of not clinging to our opinions. As Buddhist scholar Maurice Walsh wrote in the introduction to his translation of the Buddha's teachings in the Pali Canon, "It is not . . . in the true spirit of Buddhism to adopt a 'fundamentalist' attitude towards the scriptures." Even if the Buddha's method of meditation was recorded in exacting detail and was *unmistakably* clear (which it's not), we shouldn't become sanctimonious about it.

It's good to remember that the origin of a meditation technique isn't nearly as significant as its effectiveness. If the sensation-based vipassana technique presented in this book had been developed by Mr. Peabody of Des Moines, Iowa, in 1953, it would still be worthwhile—especially if we knew that Mr. P. was an uncommonly wise person who had tried many other techniques (as the Buddha had) and that his method had benefited millions of people.

Given those disclaimers, why even consider if this is how the Buddha actually meditated? Essentially, for the same reason every form of Buddhism wants to be associated with its source: for the credibility and the confidence that you're on the right track. As the British monk Ajahn Sucitto pointed out, "Meditation is the leading edge. But you need right view to know where to apply that. And certainly right view is enhanced by some accurate study. So you owe it to yourself to go back to the Buddha. You'd be foolish not to try to get as close as you can to the Master."

If someone told you that the Buddha himself was here—the real McCoy!—and he's giving a 10-day seminar on how to meditate, you'd probably rearrange your life so you could make it. Well, according to that very man who we'd be so excited to meet, it wasn't his person that was important, but what he taught. Following his genuine teachings is like getting direct instructions from him. Of course, it's not truly the same thing, but you can see the value of knowing or at least investigating what he actual taught. If we're to take the Buddha's path, it makes sense to check if our map is accurate. Still, even as I make the case that this method of meditation is how the Buddha would want us to practice, please keep the disclaimers in mind, as my intention is to present this with a light touch.

LOOKING AT THE RECORD

The basis for staking claims about the Buddha's meditation method comes from the Pali Canon. According to tradition, after the Buddha died, a large gathering of enlightened, senior monks (and presumably nuns), all of whom had heard him speak many times, came together to collaborate, confirm, and memorize the exact words the Awakened One had expounded since his enlightenment. To preserve these words (alas, there was no paper back then), monks memorized them in the form of chants (which is why the text tends to be repetitive, with a sing-songy quality when chanted in Pali). After this initial meeting of monks, other meetings would convene to make sure the Buddha's original words hadn't been altered. This went on for roughly 500 years until it was finally all written down—creating the Pali Canon that we know today.

Research shows that not all of the Pali Canon was created immediately after the Buddha's death; some of it was added over the course of many years. Still, there is wide agreement among Buddhist scholars that this sacred text is the closest record we have of what the Buddha actually taught. And while Pali scholars may disagree on the translations of particular phrasing, there is wide agreement that the discourse on awareness, known as the Satipatthana Sutta, is an accurate rendering of the Buddha's words.

The Satipatthana Sutta, which is often also called "the four foundations of mindfulness," is so important because various vipassana traditions use it to establish their meditation practices. The Satipatthana Sutta, however, isn't just about meditation; it's advice about establishing and maintaining awareness in all situations. The "four foundations" refer to the four fundamental types of human experience: our physical processes, the basic quality of an experience (pleasant, unpleasant, or neutral), moods, and thoughts. This awareness discourse is detailed in some parts (and often repetitive), yet it isn't so precise or unequivocal that there is no room for interpretation. Not surprisingly, within that interpretative space, various schools of vipassana meditation have developed.

Before focusing on differences between various vipassana traditions, however, I'd like to highlight a few points about *technique* (most forms of Buddhism agree on the basics) that the various types of vipassana do agree upon: First, the Buddha made clear that the method of mindfulness meditation which he explains in the Satipatthana Sutta is *the*, or certainly his, way for attaining enlightenment. Most translations quote him saying, "There is, monks, this *one* way to the purification of beings, for the overcoming of sorrow and distress, for the gaining of the right path, for the realization of Nirvana" (italics added). A few translators have taken "this one way" to mean, "the most direct route," or in the hands of one ecumenical translator, "this way that leads only to the purification. . . ." Regardless of which phrasing you choose (and keeping with a broad-minded spirit, let's stick with the most inclusive one), this indicates (about as definitively as possible for something which happened so long ago) that the advice he gives in the Satipatthana Sutta is how the Buddha himself meditated and how he taught other serious practitioners to as well.

It's also clear from the text that the Buddha emphasized an awareness-based meditation technique, as opposed to one that stressed concentrating on a single object, thought, feeling, or phrase. Single-focus methods had been widely taught by other gurus in India during the Buddha's lifetime, and before discovering his method, he had mastered several concentration techniques himself and recognized their value. But ultimately he saw they couldn't totally purify his mind or take him to his final goal of complete peacefulness.

A few other points about technique which all vipassana traditions agree upon are that one's meditation practice should begin with mindfulness of breathing and that, regardless of what one is aware of, you should always try to be equanimous and cognizant of the rising and passing nature of all phenomenon. This element of impermanence—which the Buddha emphasized again and again (and again) in all his teachings, as well as in the Satipatthana Sutta—point to the importance of focusing on sensations. As our awareness develops, the fleeting nature of

sensations becomes unmistakable. Sensations reveal impermanence more vividly than our other kinds of experience do.

Some types of vipassana advocate never venturing away
from our breath; that is, focusing on the breath is the only meditation technique one ever uses. Other schools add practices such
as formal walking meditation, focusing on feelings, mood, and
thoughts as objects of meditation, and using the technique of
"noting" (as in saying to yourself "thought" when noticing you
have a thought or "touching" when your foot contacts the
ground when walking). There are many other, often slight variations of these methods practiced throughout Southeast Asia and
elsewhere, but it's not necessary to detail all the different
approaches since there is essentially one significant difference
between these approaches and what Mr. Goenka teaches.
Namely, the importance one places on bringing awareness to our
actual feelings or sensations.

If we don't focus on sensations, then the Buddha's instructions in the Satipatthana Sutta don't really make sense in light of
what he taught elsewhere in the Pali Canon. The Buddha consistently and emphatically spoke of the problems caused by concepts and ideas. As the monk, Buddhist scholar, and Pali
translator, Bhikkhu Bodhi wrote in an introduction to a recent
translation of the Canon: "The Buddha teaches that the craving
and clinging that hold us in bondage are sustained by a network
of 'conceivings'—deluded views, conceits, and suppositions that
the mind fabricates by an internal process of mental commentary
or 'proliferation' and then projects out upon the world, taking
them to possess objective validity."

If that's true, then it seems unlikely that the Buddha wanted
us to deliberately comment to ourselves, however briefly, on our
activities rather than trying to observe ourselves wordlessly and
nonconceptually. Having the thought "I am frustrated" or even
noting "frustration" includes assumptions and a kind of framing
of experience. Even simple thoughts create a kind of projected,

imagined reality. Such thoughts entail a "cruder" awareness than what is needed to pick up the actual sensations that comprise frustration. The thought "frustration" doesn't give unfiltered insight into the actuality of the moment *as it is*. It doesn't make evident that there is no self and that everything is constantly changing, fundamental facts the Buddha wanted us to know. If instead of thinking "frustration," we observed a burning, dancing, or trembling sensation, we get a direct experience of flux and insubstantiality.

Also, when we say "frustration" instead of paying direct attention to what we're actually feeling, even as we say the words, we continue to react, if only subtly, to the sensations leading us to feel frustrated. That reaction causes us to be dissatisfied. Upon the Buddha's enlightenment, he gained a deep insight into what is now called the chain of dependent origination, the interwoven cycle of cognitive processing that keeps us bound to unhappiness. He saw there was only one exit route, only one way to break that chain, and that was by not reacting. Everything else on the chain was automatic and inexorable once the process started.

Sensations offer an escape hatch. Since they are the link between the physical and the mental, sensations are the only common "ingredient" in all of the four basic types of experience we have. As the Buddha said: "Everything that arises in the mind flows together with sensations." So being aware of our actual feelings lets us be directly aware, in a nonconceptual way, of every type of experience we have—including our thoughts. A trained and disciplined mind can both be aware of thoughts and the feeling aspect of those thoughts at the same time in a detached way, but for most of us, if we don't want to be pulled into the drama of our thoughts, it's much easier to stay aware of its associated sensations. This makes sensation-based vipassana especially well suited for laypeople.

My point isn't to criticize any other method of meditation, but to underscore the value of this one and consider it in a context of the Buddha's teachings—keeping in mind that no matter how valuable any method is, we shouldn't cling to it. Remember, the Buddha considered his methods to be a raft to be discarded once we reached the shore beyond mind and matter. While it's wise to choose as good a craft as possible until we make that crossing, little is to be gained by arguing about seafaring techniques. Better to be out on the water, learning how to handle the waves.

It's worth noting that one of the reasons the Buddha's original method was almost lost is that monks spent so much time memorizing his words and engaging in philosophical debates, their meditation flagged. The real work is inside us. If we truly want to find out what the Buddha meant, that's where we need to focus.

PART 3

ETHICS:
THE GOOD IN
THE GOOD LIFE

ost Westerners drawn to the Buddha's teachings are
well-educated sorts with a post-Darwinian cultural
outlook that regards moral values as largely arbitrary. This orientation, combined with the doctrineless influence
Zen has had on the West, has left many to underestimate the
crucial role ethics plays in the Buddha's prescription to heal
ourselves.

This is unfortunate since the Buddha considered morality
the foundation of spiritual practice. It's also ironic, knowing
what we now know about evolutionary science: our sense of
ethics isn't arbitrary at all, but a deeply ingrained part of our
psyche. Regardless of whether or not we believe that our ethical
sense comes from absolute commandments passed down from
above, if we ignore our moral sensitivities and squash feelings of
compassion, inevitably we suffer.

To appreciate why disregarding our inborn sense of right
and wrong builds unconscious tension—a knotting process

which constricts our awareness and in essence creates our karma—it's helpful to understand some of the biological mechanisms involved. Once we know these details, it's easier to see why paying attention to our bodily sensations with equanimity can release accumulated stress and lead to uncommon insight and contentment.

Then, with these understandings in tow, we're prepared to take the Buddha's precepts seriously. We're also better able to interpret those precepts in ambiguous situations. For no rule, including those offered by the Buddha, can perfectly apply to every situation. But if we get the spirit of the precepts, they can give guidance for almost any circumstance.

CHAPTER 10

THE MORAL ANIMAL

Origin of man now proved. He who understands baboon would do more toward metaphysics than Locke.
—*Charles Darwin,* The M Notebook

The arch battle in the universe is always: evolution versus egocentrism. The evolutionary drive to produce greater depth is synonymous with the drive to overcome egocentrism, to find wider and deeper wholes, to unfold greater and greater unions. A molecule overcomes the egocentrism of an atom. A cell overcomes the egocentrism of a molecule. And nowhere is this trend more obvious than in human development itself.
—*Ken Wilber,* A Brief History of Everything

The Greek philosopher Plotinus observed that "mankind is poised midway between the gods and the beasts." We are pulled in different directions, drawn to wisdom one moment and shoving aside a competitor the next. Over the centuries, countless theories have tried to account for this dichotomy, but none has been more compelling that Darwin's theory of evolution. Essentially, Darwin, and the scientists who've followed in his wake, tells us that our mind and body have been jerry-built over the millennia, "designed" through the push and pull of survival and competition—for food, resources, and passing on genes.

Although we are the product of competition, this doesn't make us purely selfish and competitive creatures. Traits tend to get passed on for their effectiveness, and often it's advantageous to work cooperatively. Most complex organisms in fact survive only with the help of other creatures. Our intestinal tract, for example, relies on parasites to function properly. In fact, the closer you look, the harder it is to decide whether self-interest or cooperation is more important to evolution. It seems an undercurrent of tension between the two is likely to be with us for a long time.

According to evolutionary biologists, our genetic makeup is the same as our Paleolithic ancestors who lived 40,000 years ago in small, hunter-gatherer groups—a social structure inherited in turn from their primate predecessors. In other words, our social instincts go way back. Keeping that social context in mind can illuminate how jealousy, gossip, status consciousness, and self-deception can coexist along with altruism, good will, and love.

Let's, briefly, consider the smarmy, manipulative qualities first. It's easy to see how maintaining a high status in your group improved your comfort, food, and especially mating opportunities. One way to get that status is through self-promotion, and yes, sometimes deceit. Yet if you're discovered to be an exploiter or consistent liar, your reputation is likely to drop precipitously; so it's helpful if we mask our dishonorable intentions. There's no better way to do this than by fooling ourselves about our own motivations. Then we can convincingly maintain our good intentions and innocence without advertising hidden agendas. This is why we're naturally unaware of many of our own motives. "But," as Steven Pinker, professor of cognitive neuroscience at MIT, notes in *How the Mind Works*, "the truth is useful, so it should be registered somewhere in the mind, walled off from the parts that interact with other people." This "somewhere" is felt in our body: whenever we lie, cheat, or manipulate others, on some level we register that.

Of course, it's not just unseemly traits that are helpful for survival and gene-kiting, forming alliances cemented by friendship and love come in awfully handy too. Without the bonds of love, no one would survive infancy; even few adults could survive without the help of friends or relatives in the environment our ancestors lived in.

Presented in this light, it all sounds so cynical. And it's easy to see how Darwin's one-two punch of first replacing the biblical explanation of creation and then undermining our belief in absolute morality could damage traditional religious values and leave one jaded. Indeed, it appears as though Darwin's insights, along with other scientific discoveries, are largely responsible for the powerful undercurrents of cynicism washing through the world today.

It seems, though, that this disappointment is a misunderstanding underwritten by expectations about what *ought* to be instead of accepting what is. For even if our sense of right and wrong is only functional, even if you can't come up with any absolute or philosophically elegant reasons for being moral and nice, disregarding our innate ethical instincts still hurts both ourselves and others. If cynicism was really on to something, it wouldn't feel so bankrupt and just plain lousy. What the Buddha has shown is that our best instincts need to be respected, but at the same time held lightly. Don't get all high and mighty when others make moral transgressions, but if you want to be happy yourself, you must heed your ethical instincts, or pay a price.

It's curious that one rarely hears the Buddha's and Darwin's insights mentioned together—despite the naturalist's ideas adding clarity to the Buddha's teachings and the Buddha's methods offering a rich yet unsentimental prescription for those who see themselves occupying an indifferent universe. (Certainly each pioneer, in his own field, ranks among the greatest objective observers in history.) My guess is, few bring the two together because Darwin's discovery initially looks bad for spirituality. After all, at first glance it appears as though a nod to our base instincts—our selfishness—leaves little hope for genuine wisdom, and that compassion seems out of place in a survival of the fittest world. But neither is true. Here's why:

For starters, as social animals, our cooperative instincts are very powerful. Altruism (at least within a species) is an innate, genetically programmed trait which is in everyone's best interest. In hunter-gathering days, this was abundantly clear: not only was hunting easier as a group effort, but meat wouldn't keep; it made sense to divide the bounty before it spoiled. Also, by sharing, everyone improved their odds of staying well fed; your lean times could be smoothed over with assistance from your comrades, and vice versa. Throughout the world, hunting and foraging peoples have strong sharing ethics and cultures. Sharing is simply a given. In a developed economy (and thus culture), from a entirely practical vantage point, sharing is no longer so obviously in our best interest. Yet the genetic impulse to share is still there.

When our social instincts were formed, there weren't that many of us around. We were all cousins. Even if we fast-forward to tens of thousands of years *after* we stopped genetically evolving, we were still nearly all related. As novelist and philosopher Charles Johnson wrote, "If you went back to A.D. 700, everyone on earth had a common ancestor; no two persons, regardless of their race, could be less closely related than fiftieth cousins." So sharing and altruism feels right and selfishness wrong. If you doubt it, pay attention next time you're decidedly selfish. That tension is real. Research shows that people who do regular hands-on, face-to-face volunteer work live longer and are in better general health than non-volunteering sorts. Considered as a group, the health difference between those who volunteer and those who don't is greater than the difference between smokers and non-smokers.

It's true that the Buddha went beyond ordinary, you-scratch-my-back-I'll-scratch-yours altruism. His enlightenment led him to compassion for all beings, a universal love. He discovered there actually is no self to protect, and that self-interested thinking ultimately is harmful. How can that insight be reconciled with our selfish impulses? The short answer is that the Buddha, and countless others with transcendent wisdom, have seen through the veil of our base instincts. Self-protecting instincts do exist, but they are deceptive. An instinct to protect a self doesn't mean a self truly exists any more than a dog's impulse to mark his boundaries means he's watering territory he really owns. Some instincts could be seen as delusions that are good for survival and gene replication, but bad for seeing the truth. Einstein referred to our sense of self as an "optical delusion" which causes us to fundamentally misinterpret reality. As any judge can tell you, self-interest is bad for objectivity.

It's important to remember that our instincts don't always imply how we should live. What most saliently gets passed on from generation to generation are qualities that improve a gene's chance to replicate. The result is a creature "designed" for survival and reproducing, but in our case with the potential to be so much more. Some of the biological tools we inherit, which can be seen as solely functional, also give us the capacity to find truth and peacefulness.

We all regularly transcend shortsighted impulses by appealing to a greater wisdom. For instance, despite the impulse, we don't club someone who cuts in front of us in line. And an urge to procreate doesn't imply we should sire as many children as possible. Intelligence and awareness offer options. To quote Steven Pinker's *How the Mind Works* again: "The mind is a neural computer, fitted by natural selection with combinational algorithms for causal and probabilistic reasoning about plants, animals, objects, and people. It is driven by goal states that served biological fitness in ancestral environments, such as food, sex, safety, parenthood, friendship, status, and knowledge. That toolbox, however, can be used to assemble Sunday afternoon projects of dubious adaptive value." Pinker's sentiments (minus the dubious part) could also be applied to pursuing spiritual insight and inner peace.

If one were to speculate, which admittedly the Buddha saw as a distraction from the path, one could even make a case that evolution ultimately leads to creatures who recognize the emptiness of mere survival. Noted biologists such as William D. Hamilton and Edward O. Wilson believe that once life forms developed, it was likely that some complex organisms (not necessarily in human form) would develop intelligence and self-awareness. This doesn't *necessarily* mean a hidden hand is directing things; the end result of intelligence can come from natural selection forcing a kind of ongoing arms race between species.

The basic push toward sophistication comes because as a species develops sophisticated weapons and defenses, its predators and prey must evolve too or face extinction. Given enough time and constant threats from other species, which are necessary ingredients to evolution, eventually *the* most sophisticated creature natural selection could possibly create should emerge. Knowing intelligence is possible, it seems inevitable that some species had to develop it. Once so fortified, it also seems inevitable that someone, a least one individual of the billions that pass through, would see through the whole existential setup—including their own instincts/proclivities. The incredibly long trail that leads to creatures able to transcend a purely survival mode is so awesome that missing that opportunity by focusing on satisfying our instinctual needs seems like an incredible waste.

The Buddha never denied that greed, desire, and self-interest exist. So deciphering where those impulses come from doesn't change his prescription of how to *skillfully* handle them. We simply get a deeper respect for their power. As Robert Wright wrote in *The Moral Animal,* "Many of our impulses are, by design, very strong. . . . It is grossly misleading to talk as if self-restraint is as easy as punching a channel on the remote control." By acknowledging the force of instincts, we can be clear-eyed about what we're up against. For we can't change what we don't recognize as real. Once we at least know we're wearing self-oriented-colored glasses, we can try to adjust for them. The conditioning we're seeking to undo goes way back. To find lasting contentment and transcendence of instinctual tethers, we must be prepared to make a great effort. Our inclination for a quick fix tends to undermine this necessary long-term commitment.

By recognizing and accounting for our instincts, we can defuse their power somewhat. Seeing the extent to which our problems are universal and impersonal reminds us that our own dramas aren't as exclusive or compelling as we might normally believe. Should someone insult us, for example, we may avoid getting embroiled in self-righteous scenarios for revenge if we recognize that our angry feelings are simply an instinctual response. In general, knowing we tend to be incensed or aroused after certain biological buttons are pushed indicates we should take our reactions, rationalizations, and justifications with a dose of skepticism. The point isn't to try and rid ourselves of our instincts, but to not be at their mercy.

CHAPTER 11

KARMIC ACCOUNTING AND
THE UNCONSCIOUS

*One does not become enlightened by imaging figures of light,
but by making the darkness conscious.*
—*CG Jung*

While Darwin's theory can inform our moral situation in the broadest sense, it doesn't tell us much about our individual circumstances. Why is life unfolding the way it is for us? How do our ethical choices affect our state of mind? And why can two people witness the same event at the same time yet react so differently? The Buddha taught that these are the result of our karma, the fruit of our actions and intentions. To truly understand what this means—to recognize that karma is not a quaint Eastern notion, but an inexorable law—requires a sophisticated understanding.

Usually, developing a profound appreciation of karma requires years of meditating, cultivating compassionate thoughts, and ethical behavior, but by making use of some scientific discoveries (both recent and from the distant past) it's possible for most anyone to get a good basic sense of why karmic law rules, how to understand its subtleties, and how we can align ourselves with those forces for greater peace of mind.

So let's begin as simply as possible, guided by a fundamental scientific principle: Newton's third law of motion. Sir Isaac informed us that for every action there is an equal and opposite reaction. An equation, science writer K.C. Cole explains, which "applies to all forces human and cosmic and mechanical." Clearly then, this principle should apply to our emotional reactions too. And indeed it does: each time we respond to something—anything—whether recoiling or clutching, nudging away or leaning towards, our response creates an effect.

These repercussions are important. Ultimately it means every desire, every volition, every action and reaction we have, has consequences—not because an omniscient observer is watching our every move, but by the strength of the experience itself.

It's just emotional physics: whenever we react to something, the force of that response pushes inward and outward, forward and back, influencing our present and future state of mind, and leaving an imprint that becomes part of our "past." The net result of these reactions is tension, however slight, which accumulates inside us and creates the terrain of our inner life. By understanding how this happens, we get insight into how to heal ourselves.

At the simplest level, we can notice Newton's law at work by observing ourselves if we spread nasty gossip: immediately we feel mean and ugly ourselves. It's clear that any fire we throw outward also burns us too. We cannot *consciously* harm someone else or have an unwholesome intention without hurting ourselves as well. This is the essence of karma. It's a bi-directional golden rule: by being compassionate to others, we're also being compassionate to ourselves, and vice versa. Simple as that sounds, truly living according to this principle can make an enormous difference.

Yet if we only grasp karma at this immediate level, we're likely to underestimate what we're contending with and be more likely to abandon our move toward greater kindness and awareness. But if we appreciate the nuances involved, the elements which are beyond our control, and how an effective awareness practice works in relation to these, we'll see the importance of cumulative effort. This will help us stick with the program, which will indeed yield the spiritual results we're after, and that in turn naturally reinforces our efforts. Then, we'll come to see the necessity of heeding karmic law by cultivating an equanimous awareness and thoughts which wish others well. The Buddha taught that to understand karma is to recognize the mind's role in creating—or undoing—our own unhappiness.

Karma has often been misunderstood in the West to mean one's fate or destiny. Usually it's invoked after something goes wrong: maybe we followed a stock tip and lost a bunch of money, or we fell in a pothole and broke our wrist. "I guess it's my karma," we sigh. In that resignation is a hazy sense of responsibility mixed with a nod to a higher power. Well, the vague accountability may be right; our actions do affect our life's circumstances. But to focus on material results is to focus on the most superficial aspect of karma—the part that may be beyond our control, and impossible to trace. After all, if the investment had broken even or the pothole was filled in (which of course were possibilities), our life wouldn't have changed much.

What the Buddha really wanted us to recognize is how our psycho-spiritual fate is affected by our intentions and reactions. This is an inexorable process, but often so subtle it can be difficult to recognize. As vipassana teacher and psychiatrist Paul Fleischman noted in *Karma and Chaos*, "the concept of kamma [that's Pali for "karma"] has not fit easily into Western thought, since it expresses the unity of two elements: choice and necessity. Kamma is neither freedom nor determinism, as it has been often misread to be, but a dynamic fusion of these two...."

To better understand what the Buddha meant by karma, we must admit complexity to the Newtonian world. For while his equal-and-opposite law works beautifully for describing a single incident of force, its relevance fades when multiple effects and influences are added. Obviously, we don't live in a tidy cause-and-effect, "billiard ball" universe where Newton's rules rule. Even on a pool table, if a ball flies over the side rail, the accuracy of his equations similarly fall by the wayside.

An event in our life isn't an isolated thing, but one moment in a longer, continual movement which flows like a river. Newton's law would aptly apply to any single wave or experience in that river, but that wave/moment doesn't stand alone. It is created by the wave behind it and the one behind that one and everything upstream from those. It's also affected by the new wave starting to form.

So imagine you're floating on a river. Sometimes the water flows smoothly and sometimes it's choppy. Sometimes the scenery along the shore is lovely and other times it's trashed from garbage both you and others have left. How you respond to these conditions greatly influences what the river will look like downstream. If you figure the river is already ruined and throw more garbage in, it will only get worse. If you react to rough water by flailing about, the waves will only get bigger. And if you focus mainly on fixing things along the bank, you're unlikely to notice changes in the current and how your shoreline ambitions are affecting your water quality.

Keeping the river and a fluid sense of causality in mind, we can start to make sense of an age-old puzzle: if it's true that we reap what we sow, why don't nice guys finish first in business, love, and health? Or, similarly, how come evil people and bad deeds aren't always punished? When we see that what is most meaningful in life is our state of mind or the flow and quality of our water—and not so much what's happening along the banks or in our life circumstances—we can intuit the answer. Our internal actions and intentions over a lifetime (or, according to the Buddha, lifetime*s*) always affect our waters, but what happens on the shore is affected by people and events that may be beyond our control (though many Buddhists believe the external circumstances of our life are also the result of our intentions and actions). While tracing or predicting *measurable* results from any given action, even a powerful one, is just too complex, it is still possible to learn valuable lessons from understanding a bit of river science and dynamics, which can help us learn how to surf and care for our water's quality.

To make the workings of a fluid, nonlinear and internal-focused causality more real, consider some concrete examples. Suppose, for instance, someone asks George if he ever thought about cheating on his taxes. If George says "no" and that's a lie, that creates a little bit of internal tension, a physical event that can be detected with instruments like a polygraph or brainwave machine. Should George go further and actually fudge his taxes, that action would create even more stress, though he might hardly notice it, especially after a few days passed or particularly after a few years had gone by— unless the IRS calls letting him know he's being audited.

The odds are, though, that George is likely to get away with his small fudging. So let's pretend that he decides to push the envelop and take outrageous write-offs—eventually evading all taxes by not filing at all. Clearly he's set up a dangerous situation, and lots of stress. Even if the IRS is asleep at the wheel and never notices, George will still pay a psychological price. After watching a *Law and Order* episode on a tax fraud, for example, he may be awake for nights. His fear of the IRS may become so intense, he ends up fleeing the country.

And to follow this example to completion, if George ended up strangling the IRS agent who eventually nabs him, he's unlikely to ever escape the twisted tension that murder creates, even if he eludes capture. He'll forever be on edge, close to it, or be so numbed his whole life will suffer.

KARMIC UNCONSCIOUS

While rivers and tax cheats can offer an intuitive feeling for how our actions reverberate and affect us, they don't offer a very Western way to think about psychodynamics. So unless we translate the mechanisms involved into familiar psychosomatic terms and show biological correlates, one might still think of karma in a fuzzy metaphorical way, missing its inescapable reality. To get this more profound understanding of karma, it's worth outlining the mind-body processes involved, starting with the idea that it's helpful to think of our karma much the way we consider our unconscious.

Psychoanalysts define the unconscious as a storehouse of unaware impulses, passions, and inaccessible memories that affect our thoughts and behavior. This is exactly the effect stress, tension, repression, and agita from our past actions, intentions, and reactions have on us too. Switching back to the metaphor of a river—except this time imaging we are the river itself (albeit a conscious one with free will)—we get a glimpse of how this works. The present state of our river is created by the waves before it (our past states of mind), the terrain of the riverbed (the interface of mind and body where our deepest, often unacknowledged feelings are held), our external life situation (the river banks), and how we react to all of these. If our past has created choppy, debris-filled waters and we're frustrated by the those waves, we'll produce even more turbulence, tension, and confusion. These disturbances will make it more difficult to see what's really going on inside us at the deepest level, creating a self-censoring effect—exactly what every psychotherapist working to change a client's patterns runs up against.

So what's the difference between Freud's unconscious and a karmic unconscious created by intention and reaction? No matter what you call it, the phenomenon itself is the same. But how we think of our unconscious affects how we work with it. In a karmic—unconscious paradigm, we see that we're contending with an ongoing, self-created—or, at very least, self-reinforced—process, not a *thing*, as the term "*the* unconscious" suggests.

When the unconscious is seen as a thing, it seems inaccessible and unchangeable, as though it were a large locked safe sitting in our living room. We may have some ideas about the contents inside, but mostly we need to accept it as a big, largely impenetrable obstacle that's always going to be there, cramping our living space. When we regard unconscious material as generated by a process, however, we recognize that it can—and will—wax and wane depending upon how we handle and observe the present. We see that our unconsciousness is maintained by unwise choices and a lack of awareness; so if we bring more light to our mind-body doings, it doesn't need to permanently exist. To do this, we must contend with our unconscious processes in the moment, aware of our ongoing part in its creation or release. This doesn't imply ignoring the past, but that by paying close attention to the present with skillful awareness, the past's hold on us will unravel naturally.

Unconscious material exists along a continuum, from easily noticed vague worries, like fears about getting laid off, to deeply buried pain and instinctual drives. While it is difficult to mark boundaries on a continuum, unconscious "material" can be thought of as held in our body (as outlined in chapter 4). So by bringing awareness to the literal feelings in our body, we can directly access our unconscious energies. While this might initially strike some as too simple to be true, remember that sensations have both a mental and somatic component; or put another way, sensations are where the mind and body meet.

Ⓠ

THE NEUROCHEMISTRY OF KARMA

Though understanding our karma as something like "accumulated unconscious body-held tension" helps translate it into Western terms, it still sounds so abstract. It doesn't give us the sense of precision and detail that many Buddhists associate with karma. Some Tibetan Buddhists, for instance, have made an art of accounting for the consequences of our intentions. This doesn't mean a Tibetan monk or geshe can tell you what the exact result of any single intention will be, but they have collectively mapped the general outcome of certain types of intentions.* For example, insensitivity to others' health problems is said to eventually bring on our own injuries, illness, or apparent physical discomfort. Or, useless talk, plans, and gossip will make it difficult for us to relax and will undermine our sense of confidence. If this is true, then there must be some actual mechanisms to explain it, most likely something taking place at the micro level.

Recent breakthroughs in neurobiology suggest how precise karmic accounting can be possible. Within the last couple decades, neuroscientists have increasingly concluded that our thoughts and feelings are recorded by/in neuropeptides, information-carrying chemical messenger molecules. While these feeling-recording molecules are primarily thought of as

---

* Again, to note what some will consider a convenient caveat, traditionally Buddhists believe this may not be always be manifest until a future lifetime.

part of our nervous system, they also interact with our endocrine and immune system, suggesting that neuropeptides are the whole-system, mind-body link the progressive medical community has sought.

Pioneering neuroscientist Candace Pert has dubbed neuropeptides "the molecules of emotions," meaning emotions in the broadest sense "to include the familiar human experiences of anger, fear, and sadness . . . but also basic sensations such as pleasure and pain, as well as the 'drive states' . . . such as hunger and thirst." These neuropeptides are stored in cells, essentially holding bits of data/feeling until they are released or change form. The biology of neuropeptides isn't neat or easy to account for (or universally accepted yet), but for our purposes, what's relevant about neuropeptides is that they record the effects of our stress and feelings, whether we're aware of it or not. The greater the force of the feeling, the greater the entry. We can think of this record as analogous to pieces of debris accumulating in the riverbed of our life: the force of an emotional response scatters chemical information which gets deposited in cells. These cells, which hold the "flavor" of our experience, are both stored in body parts and circulate throughout our whole body-mind, including our brain.

For dramatic evidence of the mind being everywhere in the body, consider the accounts of some organ transplant recipients: after getting a new kidney, heart, or liver, the organ-receiver reports having unfamiliar impulses, thoughts, and dreams as well as uncanny changes in facial expressions, musical choices, and food preferences that turn out to be reminiscent of the organ donor. After hearing this, some might try to explain it with supernatural accounting. A neuroscientist, however, is likely to chalk it up as more evidence that our memories, feelings, and mind are held throughout our body.

While doctors and the media have paid a lot of attention to how our emotions and repressed feelings affect our health, less notice has been given to how our feelings/neuropeptides affect our receptivity, awareness, and ability to learn. The neuropeptides in our body/mind change the protein composition of our cells and the sensitivity of the receptors in our nervous system. As Candace Pert explains in *Molecules of Emotion*:

> When a receptor is flooded with a ligand [i.e., when a piece of biochemical information has been transmitted], it changes the cell membrane in such a way that the probability of an electrical impulse traveling across the membrane where the receptor resides [i.e., where that information is received] is facilitated or inhibited, thereafter affecting the choice of neuronal circuitry that will be used.

In other words, like a river which has its flow and character changed by its history, so it goes for our body and mind. Our very experience of life is changed (and usually dulled) by, well, our experiences—or more precisely by how we react and interpret our experiences. This biochemical "editing" process explains on a molecular and cellular level why we tend to only see what we already know, lending credence to the spiritual saying, "When we are ready, the teacher appears." While this isn't news, once we appreciate the basic processes involved in narrowing our awareness, we can better understand how to undo it. We can also understand that if we want an unobstructed, clear view of reality, we need to free ourselves from our repressed and unconscious feelings. But before considering how to do that, it's helpful to look at one more significant factor which affects how a stored yet flowing unconscious operates.

RESONANCE IS REAL

Resonance is a physical and emotional phenomenon manifest when things resonate or get in sync. Buddhists sometimes speak of "like attracting like," but this sounds so vague and unscientific that we may not give it the attention it deserves. But when we realize physicists and mechanical engineers study resonance at a micro and macro level, we're more likely to appreciate the important yet often unregistered role it plays in our material, psychological, and social lives.

The reason resonance is an universal phenomenon is that at the micro level—subatomic, atomic, molecular—everything vibrates. These vibrations interact with and mutually affect the vibrations of other things. Though technical sorts can physically track and account for this phenomenon, we also know it intuitively. Put on some good dance tunes, and you have to move. Your whole being feels the rhythm and beat. Or notice how one person's buoyant mood can lighten up a dull party.

Two things are important to recognize about resonance. One is that the vibrations we tune into, the types of things we focus on, resonate throughout our whole life. So if you work on the floor of the New York Stock Exchange, odds are you're going to feel more stressed and materialistic, than, say, if you tend sheep. Similarly, the intentions and energy we create draws people and things with similar feelings toward us (and us toward them). So if we do a lot of good in the world, we're more likely to be surrounded by good people and have fortunate "accidents" happen to us.

What we don't usually intuitively recognize, though, is that a lot of similar energy vibrating at the same frequency can create big, chaotic, or unexpected effects. A kid swinging on the playground, for example, uses the rhythm of similar motions to soar above the schoolyard. Too many pushes, however, and the lad or lass will fly out of control. This is why soldiers break formation when crossing a bridge: to prevent the vibrations from the same pattern of thousands of steps from snapping the overpass.

This system-breaking aspect of resonance can be used to good or bad effect. Put a bunch of hooligans together and mayhem might break loose. Get a whole nation riled up to the tune of hatred and pig-headed nationalism and you get Nazi Germany and a breakdown in societal morality. Or for a positive effect, put a troubled soul amongst a loving family and he or she can break out of old patterns and begin to heal. One reason apathy is so dangerous is that it lets others set the tone of what happens to our world. Making it possible, as Margaret Mead famously noted, for a small group of people to effect large change.

To bring resonance back to unconscious/karmic formations, we need to briefly take another dip in the river analogy, dosing it with a little vibrancy. First we have to remember that the river is energetic. Nothing about it is solid—including the riverbed and the debris it holds. The molecules carrying our stress are dancing bits of energy. Knowing this, it's easy to see how one moment can send shock waves and excitement throughout the whole river, stirring up sediment and garbage and sometimes setting off a rogue wave. Let's say, for instance, that you had a bad day: your boss yelled at you, you got a flat tire on the way home, and then you squabble with your spouse. If later that evening your partner accidentally steps on your reading glasses, you might explode, showering them with a cascade of complaints—energy powered from stored, previously unresolved disputes and whatever other frustration got stirred up by the waves of anger coursing through you.

The phenomenon of one feeling or reaction evoking other feelings of a similar quality is actually always happening, but it's usually too subtle for us to notice. One of the reasons not to feed negative states of mind is that it multiplies our unhappiness.

CLEARING INVENTORY

When we wisely heed the laws of karma by generating positive states of mind and not reacting to the negative ones, the vibrant aspect of our stored stress can become a gift to help us heal. To do this, we need three basic tools: moral behavior, acceptance, and awareness. Ethical behavior, good intentions, and acceptance keep us from adding new thrash into our life and allows old deposits to surface and wash away, and awareness lets us see more clearly what's really happening allowing us to see the depths of our mind-body—and, for some, beyond.

This process becomes most apparent while meditating. When done skillfully, meditation sets the biophysics of the mind-body or the laws of karma working for us. In keeping with Newton's third law of equal and opposite reactions, when we are mostly nonreactive, energy held in neuropeptides gets released. Essentially what comes up is frustrated energy, even though it may be connected with pleasurable feelings or desires. Sometimes it's easy to identify the experience associated with the feelings that surface, but often it isn't.

This unraveling of held tension happens *roughly* on a "last in; first out" basis (LIFO accounting for those who've been exposed to any business parlance), but is so affected by resonance patterns that it's impossible to trace in a linear way. We can sense how this works by considering our dreams:* after falling asleep and becoming largely nonreactive, unconscious material from the day surfaces, informed by our past emotional history. That day's unresolved feelings arise, intermixed with

---

* While there is still no consensus about why we dream or need sleep, it's interesting to consider the importance of sleep (as opposed to just lying down) as a way to release some of the day's tensions. It's worth noting that the Buddha is said to have retired for only about 2 hours a night, and then only to rest his body.

older emotions that resonate with those feelings. Likewise, when we meditate, our most recent grievances, aggravations, and gloatings surface, mixed with past similar feelings.

These sensations/memories often snag us as they float by: we either become frustrated by the recollection, wrapped up in recreating the drama, or savor the sweetness of victory. But we can train ourselves to not react (or barely so) to these rehashings. And after these feelings pass, we're left a *bit* lighter, which is why we tend to feel better after meditating. When the Tibetan lama Chögyam Trungpa was asked, "What is it that's reborn after you die?" He answered, "Neurosis." In other words, the unprocessed unconscious energy we're still holding.

As one goes deeper in meditation, powerful feelings can arise, including some from the distant past. When new meditators come upon such uncomfortable feelings, they often want to abandon ship. But actually, reaching this point is a good sign. It shows we're releasing some deeply buried feelings. Ultimately, there's no point in running away; unless we face and accept these emotions, they won't ever truly leave and will continue to influence our life anyway. As Tibetan monk and former molecular biologist Matthieu Ricard said: "This process [of releasing old tension] can be called purification, not so much in the moral sense, but in a practical one, rather like the elimination of pollution. . . ."

We feel purer and clearer after meditating because we're less blocked by frustrated energy. Take this process to completion and lose all your accumulated tension, and you'll be fully enlightened. One way to describe an enlightened person is as someone who has lost the burden and influence of his or her unconscious hindrances. With the darkness gone, what's left is just wisdom and inherently good and shining qualities (which had been there all along, but obscured). It's not that the purifying process causes nirvana, but full realization comes when our blinders are gone. Naturally, this process doesn't happen in a simple, linear fashion. In a moment of pure insight, there may be a great release of distorting energy, just as a gash in a dam can release a huge amount of stored water. It's said that in the moments just before the Buddha became fully enlightened, countless previous lives passed before him. Talk about clearing inventory!

Our own attempts at clarity, acceptance, and purity tend to be approximations. It's very difficult to be perfectly aware and completely accepting of our feelings. So the unburdening process takes a while. As everyone knows all too well, we don't lose our flaws easily. So we shouldn't expect to sit down and shed our difficulties in a direct line to nirvana. Yet, we can notice if our mind stream is heading in the right direction. By respecting the laws of nature, as we travel the river of our life, our waters will become calmer, deeper, and cleaner. And when rough waters do come, we'll know how to surf.

CHAPTER 12

A FRESH LOOK AT THE P-WORD:
WHY ETHICAL PRECEPTS MATTER

There is a tendency in the West to dismiss the five precepts
as Sunday-school rules bound to old cultural norms that no
longer apply to our modern society, but this misses the role
that the Buddha intended for them: They are part of a course
of therapy for wounded minds. In particular, they are aimed
at curing two ailments that underlie low self-esteem:
regret and denial.
—*Thanissaro Bhikkhu*

The first noticeable sprouts of Buddha's wisdom appeared in this country in the late 1950s along with the Beat movement. Attracted to Zen Buddhism's intuitive and unorthodox wisdom, Beat luminaries such as Jack Kerouac, Alan Ginsberg, and Alan Watts shined their light on this once esoteric practice. Watts and company were tickled and intrigued by stories of Zen monks slapping each other and proclaiming you should kill the Buddha if you meet him on the road. Turned off to convention, heavy-handed sermonizing, and anything that reeked of commandments, Zen's eccentric wisdom was a balm to these alienated yet searching souls. Still smarting from the button-down and oppressive 1940s and '50s, the Beats—and their sixties counter-culture progeny—were powerfully drawn to Zen's iconoclasm, its apparent flouting of rules. What these early Zen enthusiasts largely missed, however, was that most of the monks portrayed in those stories were celibate vegetarians who followed incredibly disciplined regimes.

This early Buddhism phase or "Zen fad," as *Time* magazine called it, became intermingled with a hip sixties zeitgeist of psychedelics, free love, and an array of eclectic healing therapies often first showcased at the Easlen Institute. The person that probably best characterized this time was the charismatic, brilliant, and controversial former Tibetan lama Chögyam Trungpa.

Trungpa, who taught in the crazy wisdom tradition that dislodges one's familiar assumptions, attracted a large Western following and founded the Naropa Institute in Boulder, Colorado. During the day, the ex-monk gave dharma talks and built an enduring and far-flung spiritual organization; at night he drank, slept around, and partied hard with his students. In this climate, it's little wonder that renunciation got short shrift. The idea of following rules or keeping precepts sounded square—and for validation, you could quote Taoist sages, Zen masters, and other mystics who relied solely on their innate sensibilities as guides for wisdom.

Somehow the discipline of meditation seemed to fall into a different category than keeping precepts. Even if you didn't meditate yourself (as neither Watts or Kerouac ever seriously did), everyone was for it. It kind of smacked of tripping, dropping out, and doing your own thing, while at the same time being practical. It's actually this pragmatic part that has allowed meditation to survive and mostly thrive in the U.S. long after flower power has become a quaint or wistful memory.

Meditation is popularly seen as something concrete we can do to help ourselves. Its benefits are backed by scientific studies and it can double both as a spiritual exercise and a stress reducer. All that, and it's less expensive than going to a shrink. This gives meditation a sensible air which appeals to an American ethos of practical self-improvement without trampling on beliefs in unbridled freedom.

As Buddhist writer and former monk Stephen Batchelor points out, this pragmatic aura fits well with our technocentric response to problems. When Buddhist practitioners are asked, "What is your practice?" most tend to answer with what their meditation technique is. While obviously I believe one's choice of meditation method does matter, as Batchelor notes, "such responses reflect a widespread view that practice is essentially a matter of spiritual technique." From this perspective, ethics isn't seen as an integral part of the practice itself. Meditating for a half hour or hour a day becomes like spending time on the Stairmaster; after doing our exercise for the day, we can then get on with our life.

Naturally if asked, most meditators would know that ethical behavior is an important part of Buddhism. After all, Buddhism 101 tells us that morality is an integral part of the eightfold path. Yet somewhere in Buddhism's western landing, this crucial component to the Buddha's prescription has been so downplayed, it's almost been lost. Cultural dissonance has given a wide birth for rationalizations and some bad habits. On top of that, there's the plain fact that it's not always easy to be good (at least in the short term). Even the Buddha himself is said to have struggled with renunciation when he first started following a spiritual path. So we can be forgiven if we've missed the Buddha's emphasis on morality. At least I hope we can, since I had missed it too.

REALLY GETTING IT

Like most everyone, I've always, more or less, tried to be a nice guy and do the right thing. But until I really got S.N. Goenka's message about the value of keeping the precepts, I didn't realize the depth of the connection between my actions and spiritual progress. I first truly got it after having a vivid nightmare while at a retreat. To explain the significance of this dream, which happened during my second course, I need to give a little background about retreat rules and just a bit of slightly embarrassing personal history.

One of the policies of a S.N. Goenka course is that students shouldn't bring their own food. You're fed quite well for two meals a day, but the evening meal is very light (or only tea for old students) and no snacking is allowed. As a tall, thin guy who exercises a lot, this wasn't an easy rule for me. And I had reason to believe it hurt my ability to concentrate. Years before, I had attended a Zen retreat that had an inexperienced cook who never put out enough food. I struggled with flagging energy for most of the retreat, finding it difficult to stay awake. At subsequent Zen retreats I always took a small stash of food to supplement our official diet, and this was fine, according to their etiquette. I also did this for my first and part of my second 10-day vipassana courses, even though I knew it was against the rules. I figured I wasn't hurting anybody and kept my imported snacks hidden in rodent- and insect-proof containers. And I only snacked very discretely as not to disturb anyone else.

After meditating intensely for a few days, our access to what is normally considered our unconscious increases. This heightened awareness often even carries over to when we're sleeping, making dreams incredibly vivid. During my first two vipassana retreats, most of this nightly vibrancy took the form of disturbing dreams. At the time, though, I didn't connect the dots—until I had a particular nightmare. In this bad dream, I was lying on the ground wearing a mask and a Zen robe. The toes of each of my bare feet were arranged to form peace signs (no, I can't swing this while I'm awake). Then someone came over and ripped off the mask. I woke up in the middle of the night, startled and upset. It wasn't until later the next day that I realized that I had been pretending to be a good, peaceful Buddhist, but I was in fact *lying*. After that, I stopped snacking, never took food along again, and the bad dreams stopped.

What I finally, clearly recognized was the truth of "you can run, but you cannot hide." No one had caught me noshing, and I really wasn't hurting anyone else, but I was lying and I paid a price for it. It's the karmic law of stress: create tension and it will come back your way. Our intentions and actions have reverberations and consequences. To paraphrase Insight meditation teacher Joseph Goldstein, our only real possessions are our accumulated wholesome and unwholesome intentions.

When we act unethically, we add to our psychic burdens (or karmic debt, to use Buddhist phrasing). Once we see this, we realize if we want to be happy, we really have no choice but to try to be moral. Not because it's written in a book somewhere or because the Buddha said so, but because it's good for our own sanity and well-being, as well as everyone else's. Often we frame issues in our life as dilemmas of whether we should help ourselves or help others, be good to ourselves or nice to others. Yet this is actually a misleading setup. By being kind to others, we are being compassionate to ourselves, and vice versa. Notice how when you focus on how other people are doing, genuinely wishing them well and working for their welfare, you're in a good state of mind yourself. Enlightened self-interest is built into our very being, and it's a beautiful thing.

When we pay attention, we know in our heart when we're doing the right thing and when we're not. We know the difference between telling a white lie to protect someone's feelings, and rationalizing or cheating "just a little." That bit of cheating and laziness eats away at our integrity and peace of mind. Often it happens in such small increments, we don't recognize it. But we do notice the opposite: when we're honest and true we feel clean, fresh, and light. That is the reward of being unburdened. It's worth reflecting upon the fact that these feelings persist even in a culture that puts more emphasis on success and having fun than on goodness.

Our intuitive sense of right and wrong often gets confused by other motivations. That's why some discipline and effort devoted toward learning how to handle our feelings skillfully is important. Precepts act like guardrails, supporting our best, overall intentions at times when we're distracted and distanced from what's happening inside us. Precepts keep us from veering off the road leading to peacefulness. These guides can't take the place of intuitive wisdom, but they can help us when we're driving through a fog.

Q

THE PRECEPTS IN CONTEXT

The Buddha's five precepts (there are eight for monks, nuns, or devoted householders and ten for mendicant monks and nuns) are basic ethical guidelines that steer us toward a more satisfying life and greater purity of mind. These precepts should be considered the foundation of creating a healthier and happier existence. To quote what S.N. Goenka has said many times, "Anyone who wishes to practice Dharma [be aligned with natural laws] must begin by practicing morality. This is the first step without which we cannot advance."

Mr. Goenka is not speaking of the precepts as a literal first step in the sense that you should wait until you're ethically pure before meditating. Each aspect of Buddhist practice reinforces and strengthens the others so that they work together: we need a calm mind to deeply examine ourselves, but we can't be calm if we're agitated over something we've done wrong; similarly, when we have a serene, penetrating awareness, we can clearly see the value of ethical intelligence and so we're less tempted to behave badly. We also have a greater awareness of our real-time actions—making it less likely we'll act harmfully.

Understood in this way, we see it doesn't really make sense to devote yourself to a meditation practice without also committing yourself to being ethical. But behaving ethically means different things to different people; what exactly should it consist of?

In an essay titled "The Healing Power of the Precepts," Thanissaro Bhikkhu, the abbot at Metta Forest Monastery near San Diego, makes an articulate case for keeping precepts as simple as possible; he believes that if we make ethical guidelines particularly lofty or noble, we may set impossibly high standards and goals we're likely to fall short of, resulting in more tension for us. He points out, for instance, that those who translate the precepts "do not kill" or "do not steal" into edicts that we shouldn't harm the planet, are setting themselves an impossible task since so many of our actions leave at least traces of pollution on our hand. This isn't an argument against environmental stewardship, but one for clear-cut moral rules which, as Thanissaro Bhikkhu says, "don't allow for unspoken agendas to come sneaking in the back door of the mind. If, for example, the precept against killing allowed you to kill living beings when their presence is inconvenient, that would place your convenience on a higher level than your compassion for life. Convenience would become your unspoken standard—and as we all know, unspoken standards provide huge tracts of fertile ground for hypocrisy and denial to grow."

This is wise advice, and maintaining a strong commitment to the essential, unmistakable aspects of the precepts is important, but it doesn't mean one should interpret the precepts too narrowly either (a point, based on his other writings, I believe Thanissaro Bhikkhu would agree with). The precepts were never intended to be a rulebook which allows us to escape moral ambiguity or leave behind our innate sense of wisdom in the moment. As Zen priest Steve Hagen observed in *Buddhism Plain and Simple*, "The Buddha did not lay down any commandments. If we say, 'Thou shalt not lie,' applying it as a rule, what are we to do when the Gestapo pounds at our door and we're harboring a family of innocent fugitives in the attic?"

We must look beyond the edict of the precepts to the values and spirit they encourage. If we were to just stick literally to the precept of "do not kill," for example, but are still filled with hatred, we won't exactly thrive spiritually. We should also try to wish the best for others. One way to resolve the need to both have clear-cut guidelines and yet try to do more than just stay out of jail, is to approach the precepts the way you might caring for your body. At the minimum we need to brush our teeth, go to the doctor when we're ill, and take a walk and eat some vegetables every now and again. But if we really want to be healthy, it helps to get some vigorous exercise and consistently eat well.

The question then becomes, how can we know if the "extras" we choose are wise and aligned with what the Buddha intended or mixed with our own agendas or impossible standards?

I believe this is where it can be helpful to first remember that the Buddha's way puts us in harmony with the natural order of things, and next look to that natural order. If we recall that our moral sense was formed in a context of coexisting in a small clan, we get a sense of what to include and what to eliminate from the spirit of the precepts. In this light, keeping the baseline edicts—such as do not kill, steal, or lie—appears more urgent than ever: when our instincts were formed, killing someone or stealing something probably meant taking the life or property from a cousin, brother, or father. But we also see why just sticking to the minimum of not harming other members of our family isn't enough: hating one of them or wishing them ill would also create lots of tension. Keeping this evolutionary framework in mind, we get a better sense of how to apply the precepts to our life. We see, for example, why breaking the bonds of marriage or a commitment (which probably meant having sex with our cousin's or sibling's partner) would cause serious problems and worry. We also see why using someone sexually would clearly be a bad idea (not only would we then have to face them the next day at the office, but for the rest of our life), but that sexually abstinence wouldn't be necessary.

Understanding the precepts in this context has another advantage: it can counter our Western leanings toward guilt—something the Buddha never intended the precepts to do. Peace activist and meditation teacher Thich Nhat Hanh has actually suggested dropping the word "precepts" in favor of "mindfulness trainings." Many of his students found that trying to observe "precepts" evoked strong ideas of good and evil. If they broke a precept, they felt like failures. If this happens to you, then sure, think in terms of training guidelines. Remember that the precepts are meant to bring us peace of mind.

THE FIVE PRECEPTS

1. Do Not Kill: Clearly no one is going to argue against this; yet, even this most obvious precept (and notice that they are listed in order of importance) can lead into gray territory. Do you, for instance, eat meat? Do you swat a fly that lands on your arm? Do you support good causes, but wish your enemies harm?

Where we draw the line of care is something for each of us to figure out for ourselves. The Buddha made it clear that it's intention that matters. He never suggested, as say Jainists do, that we keep our mouth covered to avoid mistakenly swallowing an insect. We all must kill something to eat, but will it be a soybean plant or a cow? There is no requirement that Buddhists be vegetarians—and that makes sense, understood in light of evolutionary-formed instincts: eating an animal wouldn't create any obvious tension for you. But you will walk lighter if you choose tofu over beef. Eating meat requires violence and blood shed, and some believe that when you eat an animal you absorb some of its fear and anxieties.

2. Do Not Steal: Another lay-up. But if we expand the sentiment to include not taking what is not rightfully ours, we see how this can expand our compassion. How much of our lifestyle and livelihood is based on exploitation? Do we buy products that we know have been made with sweatshop labor? If we are an employer or hire contractors, do we pay fair wages or try to get the most we can for the least compensation? How about in our relationships with our employer, community, or spouse? The Buddha didn't recommend practicing right livelihood because it's politically correct, but so that we would purify our mind of negativities and diminish our self-centeredness. Approached in this way, we see what we're really talking about is generosity and greed. How closely do we clutch our possessions? How hungry are we for more? Being released from these urges is liberating, allowing generosity, love, and compassion to circulate better.

3. Sexual Misconduct: During a meditation retreat one is asked to abstain from all sexual activity. That's clear and simple enough, but once a course is over, few of the precepts are more gray than "sexual misconduct." Adultery is generally an easy one: that's out—and with good reason since it inevitably leads to deceit and a great deal of pain.

Most Buddhist teachers also advise against sexual flings; they recommend that you be in a committed relationship before having sex. Yet others wiser than myself suggest that uncommitted sexual liaisons could be acceptable if they are honest, tender, and responsible. The best golden rule I've heard is "don't let passion override compassion."

This rule could be applied—if stretched a bit—to self-pleasuring (which teachers never seem to discuss). Celibacy works well for some and is required for monks, but for most of us it creates undue tension; so sometimes it may be compassionate (to yourself) to release built-up sexual energy. The thing to watch for is whether the desire for sexual release turns into an addiction, a predatory outlook, or a fantasy life which ends up increasing our stress. As a general guideline, when flying solo, it's better if you can focus on the sensations of sex, rather than letting your fantasies run wild.

Attachment to sexual pleasure is no better or worse than attachment to money, donuts, or anything else. And hostility to sexuality—which tends to come from a strict puritanism—is like all aversion; it's fear based. It's important to remember that while the goal of the Buddha's teaching is to purify our minds, it's not a puritanical religion.

4. Abstain from False Speech: For most of us this can be the hardest precept to observe. It's very difficult to go through a whole day speaking only the truth, and harder still to only say the thoughtful or appropriate. False speech covers a broad ground. Most obvious is not telling outright lies, insulting people, or being verbally abusive. Clearly those are hurtful and bad for one's peace of mind. Beyond that are the exaggerations and white lies that make us temporarily feel good, the mistrusts of confidence we let slip, the gossiping that makes us feel cheap even as we utter the words, and speaking with a split tongue—saying one thing to one person and the opposite to another.

When I was a stockbroker, exaggerating and sometimes even lying were part of the trade—at least as I was taught. After doing this for a while, I started confusing fact and fiction in my own mind, even when I wasn't at the office. The more honest we are (and no, that isn't an excuse to be hurtful), the better our grip on reality; the more connected we are to the truth. To find truth, we need to be truthful.

Going further, skillful speech means we are being careful about what we say. Are we aware of how our tone of voice, body language, or the way we ask questions can be welcoming or insensitive and hurtful? Are our opinions thoughtful? Most of us were raised to believe we should have lots of strong opinions since they are a sign of intelligence. So we may spout off, but how carefully have we reflected on those beliefs? Or even if we have, how rigidly do we hold our convictions? It's rare that something worth having an opinion about isn't a magnet for other conflicting, intelligent views. This implies that often there may not be a right or wrong answer—or, at the very least, that the issue is complex. Before condemning or rushing to judgment, look closely at how your own discomfort may be coming into play. If we're pro-choice, for example, we may be impatient with anti-abortion activists (or vice versa) because their arguments strike an uncomfortable chord. This doesn't imply condoning all viewpoints, especially if someone is harming others, but it's possible to be against something—even strongly so—without using violent or reactive language or feelings. This even has the side benefit of making honest, genuinely held beliefs come off as reasonable and considerate.

5. Do Not Take Intoxicants: Some Western teachers have interpreted this precept to mean you shouldn't drink enough to cloud your mind. Mr. Goenka, following the letter of the fifth precept, takes it quite literally: one should refrain from all drinking, smoking, snorting, etc. His reasoning is that one drink can affect your mind and it easily leads to another and another.

Alcohol does have a creeping strength. Almost all the casual but regular drinkers I know find over the years they want more and more and more—and recognize that they have to impose some discipline or slip toward alcoholism. Why even start down that road?

If refraining from the occasional glass of wine or beer seems too restrictive for you, then at least try to be mindful of how much you drink and how it affects you. If you don't like what you see, then the choice should be obvious. But even if you decide to totally ignore this precept (assuming you're not a problem drinker), that doesn't suggest you should abandon the other training guidelines. It's better to observe even one of these precepts well than to discard them because you can't do them all perfectly. As the Buddhist nun Chan Khong said, "If you practice even one mindfulness training deeply, you will find that you are also keeping the other four, even without making a formal promise to do so. The Five Mindfulness Trainings are very much interconnected."

Going further with this precept means treating your mind-body well. Do you snack on junk food or junk media? Do you spend time with people who are sensitive and care about making themselves and the world a better place? Being thoughtful about what you ingest—in the fullest sense of the word—shows appreciation for your existence. The point isn't to become obsessive and fearful about our diets, but to respect and care for what is only partially ours (if we had total control of our mind-body then we'd never get sick or die). By taking good care of the things in our control we show a respect for everything. Like saying grace or thanks before you eat, it is a way of showing gratitude for the opportunity this life has given us.

PART 4

WISDOM:
A SUBTLE UNDERSTANDING

There's the way things are (or aren't), and then there's the way we *think* things are. Very often these don't correspond—particularly when it comes to existential matters and anything that threatens our ego or habitual way of doing things. For this reason, some aspects of the Buddha's teaching, notably selflessness, nirvana, and a "middle-way" approach to pleasure and pain can be confusing. Referencing some scientific research, however, can make it easier to understand these otherwise difficult Buddhist insights. Scientific findings can act as an impartial arbiter that neuters impulses to dismiss unfamiliar perspectives as "for mystics only."

Of course, nirvana, the Buddha's ultimate realization, is beyond science or any definitive explanation, but by placing what we know (and don't know) about nirvana in the proper context, we can still glean an understanding that informs our spiritual practice.

CHAPTER 13

NAVIGATING A MIDDLE WAY
THROUGH THE BIOCHEMISTRY OF
PLEASURE AND PAIN

---

*The essence of addiction . . . is that pleasure tends to dissipate
and leave the mind agitated, hungry for more. The idea that just
one more dollar, one more dalliance, one more rung on the
ladder will leave us feeling sated reflects a misunderstanding
about human nature—a misunderstanding, moreover, that is
built into human nature; we are designed to feel that the next
great goal will bring bliss, and the bliss is designed to evaporate
shortly after we get there. . . . As the Bible puts it, "All the labor
of man is for his mouth, and yet the appetite is not filled."*
—*Robert Wright,* The Moral Animal: Why We
Are the Way We Are; The New Science of
Evolutionary Psychology

Philosophers, sages, and scientists throughout the ages
have sought and pointed to *the* thing—that essential
force or urge that motivates us and sets the wheels of life
in motion. Aristotle, for instance, proclaimed it was happiness;
Darwin, the quest for survival and offspring; Freud, sex. For the
moment, let's not worry about the nuances of these theories,
who actually got it right, how these ideas fit together, or whether
they contradict each other. For there is something that every
powerful motivator has in common: how they get us to do their
bidding.

Pleasure and pain. Pain and pleasure. These are the essential binary options of nature's operating system. With just these two prods, it's possible to motivate an infinite variety of creatures. Give a lizard pangs of hunger, and off it goes in search of bugs. Or, make mating a good time (for at least one of the parties involved), and behold, Generation B keeps the flame burning until we get a Gen X. A pleasure/pain or approach/retreat mechanism is necessary for survival and passing on genes. It's a biological law, hardwired into our beings. And it makes sense that this mechanism should work in a nonverbal, sensation-based way—so both a baby and a beaver can respond.

So simple. Yet so powerful. Empires, fiefdoms, and life after life after life are spent pursuing the siren call of pleasure and attempting to skirt the shoals of pain. No one had to teach us this. We've sought pleasure and struggled against pain from birth. And little changes as the years unfold—except the ways we seek pleasure and try to avoid pain become more sophisticated, though still largely unconscious. These unconscious responses, repeated again and again, create the patterns and contours of our psyche.

Recognizing the power of the pleasure principle isn't exactly headline news. Even if Freud hadn't considered it the mind's organizing principle, it doesn't take a Ph.D. in introspection to know pleasure and pain have a grip on us. What casual contemplation is likely to miss, however, is the astonishing depth of that grip. Our every sensation, emotion, and idea—including our most profound thoughts and scarcely detectable feelings— carry the flavor of pleasure and/or pain. Even so-called neutral feelings contain hints of them.

The question is, how can we learn to work skillfully with pleasure and pain so they don't derail our efforts toward genuine contentment? The full answer to this is newsworthy, since it's been either largely overlooked or misunderstand for centuries. Freud never found a truly satisfying way to work with pleasure and pain; the best he could offer his clients, even after successful therapy, was "ordinary *un*happiness." Like most Westerners, it didn't occur to him that our very approach to pleasure and pain—trying to hold on to the former and keep the latter at bay—causes dissatisfaction.

Even recognizing that craving causes suffering doesn't necessarily lead the way to a clear solution. When Siddhartha Gautama was a seeker, it was common knowledge among spiritual teachers in India that craving was the source of our disease. The trouble was (and still is) eliminating that craving. One school of yogis Gautama followed—in the tradition of religious zealots with flogging tendencies the world over—turned to brute force, trying to bludgeon craving out of themselves.

Before developing "The Middle Way," Siddhartha experimented with extreme asceticism, fasting for months, holding his breath till he had pounding headaches, and meditating surrounded by a circle of fire under the hot, midday sun. While this regime must have improved his self-discipline and concentration, the more noticeable result was that it turned him into a decrepit skeleton (Gautama was no slacker): not only had the punishments and self-denial not destroyed his desires, if anything, they were stronger than ever since he was so deprived. Realizing you can't stomp out pleasure and pain, Siddhartha abandoned asceticism.

To a modern ear, Gautama's asceticism seems like an obvious perversion of a spiritual practice. But when you understand that craving causes unhappiness, devising a healthier alternative isn't so simple. Most everyone who takes the Buddha's path seriously has, at some point, put themselves in opposition to pleasure. Instead of just observing it, we feel we must resist it, thinking of pleasure as bad in some way.

Of course, the vast majority of people have the opposite problem: they don't want to let go of pleasure. To counter this, especially in the pleasure-centric West, Buddhist teachers often talk about the value of renunciation. Sometimes listeners interpret this to mean pleasure is bad or unwanted. But it's not pleasure itself that's the trouble, but our response to pleasure. Pleasurable feelings can actually be important indicators. After all, how would we know we were heading in the right direction unless it made us feel better? If taking the Buddha's advice made us feel generally worse, it wouldn't make much sense. Pain, suffering, and dissatisfaction are the starting point of the Buddha's path; pain lets us know something is wrong and that we need to do something different.

What we need is a discerning and sophisticated approach to pleasure, pain, and their offspring, neutral sensations. In a way, Buddhism can be boiled down to learning how to handle these three wisely. The emphasis in each of the three fundamental aspects of Buddhist training—awareness, compassion, and wisdom—corresponds to the ways we misinterpret pleasure, pain, and neutral feelings. Grasping for pleasure, pushing away pain, and misunderstanding neutral sensations are the sources of greed, hatred, and delusion.

For many Westerners, words like "greed" and "delusion" sound harsh. They echo of puritanism and mingle uncomfortably with notions we carry about sin. Knowing also that in some traditions Buddhist monks and nuns are supposed to avoid "sense pleasures" like movies and music can reinforce that confusion and create a sense of burden. It's important to remember, though, that when practiced correctly, Buddhism has, at most, a light touch. That doesn't mean it's easy or that we can avoid pain and the hard stuff, but the approach itself shouldn't feel burdensome. Since the Buddha's path heads us toward freedom, if following it feels oppressive, odds are we're doing something wrong.

Understanding nature's "intent" through scientific research on pleasure and pain can help shed light on the Buddha's guidance—while neutering our tendency to misconstrue his advice that has potentially heavy religious overtones. By learning, for example, that the neurochemistry of pleasure and addiction is essentially the same, we can understand how pleasure can be problematic if not handled with good judgment. While combining the Buddha's insights with science's, we won't end up with a simple formula, but we'll have a better chance to proceed as the Buddha intended us to.

THE BIOCHEMICAL BASICS OF PLEASURE

Our nervous system—the network in our body responsible for feeling and consciousness—is made up of neurons (cells which make up and connect our nerves, spinal column, and brain) which communicate with each other through neurotransmitters (chemicals which transmit nerve impulses across synapses). The information in and composition of these neurotransmitters, affects—and is inseparable from—our very experience of life. Thanks to antidepressants such as Prozac, everyone now knows that altering our neurochemistry changes our moods, thoughts, and actions. What's lesser known is that Prozac's agent, serotonin, is just one of many mood-altering neurotransmitters. Inside us is a sophisticated and diverse apothecary of powerful endogenous "drugs," capable of changing how the world appears.

Many chemicals in our nervous system wear different hats. Depending upon the neurochemical situation/mix, the same neurotransmitter can produce a variety of feelings and behaviors. And any single action or emotion releases many combinations of neurochemicals which lead to both direct and diffuse chain reactions. For our purposes, however, we'll mostly focus on the two prime neurotransmitters responsible for pleasure: dopamine and opioids (better known as endorphins).

There's really only one important anatomical fact we need to remember about dopamine: it is located primarily in the brain areas connected with planning, judgment, and emotion. The biological function of the dopamine system is to set priorities by rewarding behaviors it deems useful for survival and reproduction. (It's no accident that eating and sex feel good.) Working as a positive reinforcement, the release of dopamine helps us remember what to approach and what to avoid, playing an important role in how we learn. Essentially, if something feels good, dopamine was released (or, as in the case of cocaine use, made to hang around longer than usual). Usually we think a recreational drug causes pleasure, but actually it's that the drug is just stoking our dopamine pathway in some way. Not surprisingly, this "pleasure pathway" as neuroscientists have dubbed the dopamine network, is linked to all forms of addictive behavior, from heroin to gambling. Wire up a mouse, give it a lever that can electrically tickle this pleasure pathway, and the rodent will push furiously, until it drops, preferring its ecstasy to food, water, or sex.

Opioids or endorphins* produce pleasure by stimulating the release of dopamine as well as by offering their own reward. Opioid receptors and transmitters are located throughout the body, though they are concentrated mostly in the emotional centers of our brain. Opioids are chemically similar to heroin, morphine, or opium (thus the name). Not surprisingly, a surge of endorphins can lead to euphoric feelings, block pain, and be addicting.

---

* The terms, opioids and endorphins can be used interchangeably as long as one doesn't assume endorphins are restricted to causing "runner's high." Also note, there are similar, if less known endogenous opioids called enkephalins and dynorphins.

ℚ

THE BIOCHEMICAL BASICS OF PAIN

The neurochemical circuitry of pain is very complicated. There isn't one "mechanical" model that satisfies everyone. Yet, most neuroscientists conclude that there is at least one and probably two (or more) pain pathways. These pathways transmit signals (most notably via the neurotransmitter substance P) from pain receptors throughout our body to a part of the brain called the thalamus.

The thalamus does several jobs; most notably for now, it is involved with discharging instinctual reactions and acts as a relay station between emotional and cognitive parts of the brain. When the thalamus receives pain signals, it "consults" with both the emotional and analytic sections of the brain, and these help the thalamus decide how to react. These "decisions" then bring forth other biochemical responses, which effect the sensations of pain we're feeling. So if we've broken our ankle, but need to turn tail from a bear, we're flooded with adrenaline and endorphins so that we can run without feeling hurt. Or, if we slightly scrape our knee and see it's nothing serious, serotonin kicks in to calm us. In both cases, our experience of pain changes because the neurochemistry has.

What makes the molecular tracing of pain so tricky is that information can move bi-directionally along our pain pathways. Signals from the body can indicate pain to the brain, yet those "body" messages can be immediately changed by the neurochemicals the brain/our emotions responds with. Thus, the placebo effect: our beliefs and feelings can activate endorphins to prevent pain. According to a study of 500 dental patients, for example, a person receiving a placebo injection and reassurance will feel less pain on average than a patient receiving real anesthetic, but no reassurance. It's not that the duped patient is being stoical; they actually don't feel pain because they've effectively self-administered endogenous painkillers.

Similarly, though conversely, thoughts and feelings can initiate reactions in our pain pathway, causing us to feel aches and agony, even though nothing "physically" seems to be wrong. As pain specialist Dr. Don Ranney wrote, "Pain is a perception, not . . . a sensation, in the same way that vision and hearing are." Much of the unexplainable pain we feel, including some debilitating chronic pain, could be seen as something like a reverse placebo effect—pain we create. Both classic and reverse placebo effects make clear that we can't separate the emotions, preferences, and interpretations involved in an experience from the "bodily" event.

HANDLING PAIN

The interpretative aspect of pain hints at the potential for relief. If, "all pain is subjective," as the International Association for the Study of Pain concludes, then by changing how we react to painful sensations, we can change whether they are distressing.

Ultimately, pain is caused by resistance. If we decide, consciously or unconsciously, that we don't want a sensation, that sensation hurts. This is easiest to see with experiences that could be considered either desirable or painful. Pre-performance jitters, for example, could be taken either as nervousness or excitement; an adrenaline rush could either cause a panic attack or be a thrill; hot salsa tingles for some and sends others sprinting to the water cooler.

It's much harder to recognize the spin control aspect of pain when we're physically injured; the pain feels so real and inherent in the experience itself. But think of how a child and an adult might react to a slight knee scraping. Odds are the little one would bawl, while we'd just say ouch and forget about it. Of course, we're supposed to feel *something*; we're probably even supposed to be somewhat alarmed. The neuronal signals we get when tissue gets damaged is valuable information, indicating we need to tend to the injury. But it doesn't need to cause us anguish.

When we remember that our pain referee, the thalamus, is connected to instinctive responses, it makes sense that serious physical injuries would feel inherently painful, without room for interpretation. Yet a very aware and disciplined mind still wouldn't turn even these S.O.S. signals into pain. If the Buddha broke his leg, for example, of course he'd experience sensations letting him know not to put weight on it. But he wouldn't suffer. He'd be aware of the information, but you couldn't exactly call it pain.

You needn't be a spiritual master, though, to change your perception of pain. Anyone who mindfully investigates an ache instead of wishing it would leave can see that pain disintegrate. When similar awareness is applied to psychological discomfort, which is the majority of our disease, the potential for healing is tremendous.

Our psychic complexes are essentially formed and strengthened by resisting pain. When we resist feelings connected to the past, we experience anger or guilt. When we balk at feelings connected to the future, we feel anxiety. Taken collectively and mixed up in various combinations, these moments of resistance lead to distortions and dysfunction in our personality. In *Toward a Psychology of Awakening*, Buddhist-influenced clinical psychologist and psychotherapist John Welwood writes:

> We become disabled, unable to function in areas of our lives that evoke feelings we've never learned to tolerate. Turning away from this primary pain creates a second, ongoing level of suffering: living in a state of contraction and constricted awareness.

In time, these contractions form the nucleus of an overall style of avoidance and denial. We develop a whole identity, or view of ourselves, based on rejecting painful aspects of our experience. If we can't handle anger, for instance, we might try to be a "nice person" instead.

Unfortunately, as we all know, accepting painful feelings isn't so easy. And, paradoxically, it doesn't work if we're trying to make pain disappear. In a Catch-22 kind of way, it's only when we stop reacting to a feeling as if it were painful that it stops being painful. There's a subtle but significant difference between truly accepting pain and trying to make ourselves feel good or stiffly enduring it—which are still forms of resistance. Genuine acceptance not only takes a willingness to let go, but also a keen present-moment awareness.

Knowing that the Buddha advised us to accept painful feelings, some have misinterpreted this as an endorsement of passivity in the face of trouble. Yet if we remember that pain tells us something is awry, it's obvious that he couldn't have intended us to ignore it. Certainly the Buddha himself wasn't passive. Once he became enlightened he didn't ignore suffering. In fact, he became more sensitive to other's pain and devoted his life to helping. But it didn't cause him anguish. In the same way that he would know to put a splint on a broken leg yet still not suffer from the injury, he was able to attend to suffering in the world with a balanced mind, free of struggle. The implications for us are clear: while developing an accepting awareness, we shouldn't ignore pain—our own or others. When something is bothering us, we should first check in and look at the self-created aspect of the problem, but that doesn't suggest ignoring abuse and injustice. If anything, as we become less overwhelmed by our own problems, we become more sensitive to others' problems.

℗

NOT AS NEUTRAL AS THEY SEEM

Naturally, most of the time we aren't in the grips of agony or ecstasy, but just drifting along, sort of okay. What we call neutral feelings, though, still carry traces of good and bad feelings; they're just so slight we tend not to notice them.

Most people don't realize that pleasure and pain come together. Since one feeling usually dominates our awareness, we don't notice the element of pain in pleasure and vice versa. This can be easier to detect with a neutral sensation. If, for example, we have a blind date in a month, we're probably both a bit eager and a bit anxious. As the evening comes closer, we may become really nervous; yet the pleasant eager and curious parts don't totally disappear, even if the uncomfortable part overshadows it.

While the yin-yang aspect of pleasure and pain is harder to see in strong feelings, it's still there and can be observed with a sensitive awareness—or when a feeling is incredibly intense. A powerful orgasm, for example, rides the razor's edge between pleasure and pain. And sometimes when pain is so overwhelming that we stop resisting it, we find a kind of satisfying release. Biologically, it makes sense that pleasure would accompany pain; our body releases endorphins to help ameliorate our woes.

What are we to make of this inextricable connection between pleasure and pain? First, it's a reminder of the Buddha's First Noble Truth: even the best of pleasures can't give us total satisfaction. We also realize there is a good news flip side: it's possible to find a haven even while feeling the worst pain. Usually, though, we overreact to pain and pleasure—wanting to get rid of our pain immediately and never let go of feeling good. By remembering neither is permanent, or even possible to feel completely, we see the importance of maintaining a balanced mind.

Last, by knowing we always feel at least a bit of pleasure and a bit of pain, we see the need to be aware of each moment, lest we fall into delusions. Our natural tendency is to try and avoid the hard part in any moment and increase the pleasureable aspect. This means, typically, when we're not seized by pleasure or pain, we unconsciously tend to drift toward egotistical fantasies. Essentially, we try to nudge neutral feelings firmly into the pleasant and permanent column. This inclination hints at the addicting influence pleasure has on us.

TROUBLE IN PARADISE:
PROBLEMS WITH PLEASURE

When we remember that the biochemistry of pleasure is essentially the same as addiction, it's not surprising that pleasure's allure can put us on a string. Opioids are potent. Endorphins are just as addicting as heroin and morphine and some of the opioids we produce are 200 times stronger than morphine. After endorphins were discovered, doctors tried them as painkillers; the hope was that since they're produced naturally endorphins wouldn't have the addicting side effects of codeine or morphine. That wasn't true. As Dr. Robert Ornstein wrote in *The Healing Brain*, "It seems any substance that acts on the opioid receptors to relieve pain and induce pleasure is likely to be addicting."

"Addict" is a powerful label in our culture, usually reserved for those desperate from drug abuse or an obsessive behavior. So unless we're hooked on cigarettes, martinis, or gambling, we consider addiction issues to be someone else's problem. Yet looking a bit closer at our relationship to pleasure and its associated biochemistry reveals that most of us have at least a few addictive tendencies. This doesn't suggest we're pure hedonists or escapists, but that if we're not aware of the potentially addicting aspects of pleasure we're likely to fall under its sway in ways that inhibit awareness, insight, and a deeper contentment.

Full-blown addicts suffer from a type of extreme narcissism; their habit takes center stage and if they don't get their fix, they panic. Of course that kind of urgency is in a different league from liking a nightly cocktail, being hooked on sitcoms, or having a junk food jones. But we can sense the similarity when we notice how we become cranky if something derails our morning coffee or weekend plans. Much of our life is organized around our pleasures. Even our work life is often sustained by fantasies of what we'll buy with our paycheck or feel when we get the recognition we deserve—each daydream bringing hits of endorphins and dopamine. The neuroscientist Candace Pert noted that, "to some extent, we perceive the world through an opiate haze."

Pleasure's seduction can be hard to see in our own life, and we'd find it irritating if anyone else pointed it out to us. Yet, it's pretty easy to see at a societal level. Materially we're more comfortable than ever, but most folks seem more consumed with comfort than ever—at the expense of lots more important stuff. For an obvious example, corporations, stockholders, and the majority of voters consistently ignore signals from the natural environment that tell us we're living in an unhealthy and unsustainable way. Yet like the junkie, we're so entranced by our fix (more comfort and better stuff), we ignore this and other vital aspects of our collective lives.

Our economy is largely built upon satisfying desires— putting us in a more tempting context than we were designed for. Even if we have the same basic cravings as our Paleolithic ancestors, it was plainly harder for them to gratify such impulses. Our Stone-Age cousins may have dreamed of abandoned beehives full of honey, but we can just zip down to the local convenience store to grab a Milky Way bar. Easy access to an endless palette of products which promise instant satisfaction makes us more beholden to our cravings. Our carrot is never far off, so we always want one.

In chapter 2 we saw how we're distracted from our underlying discontent by the illusion that we can hop from one pleasurable moment to the next, but we didn't note how habitually doing this puts us on a cycle of increasing dependence. Those studying drug addiction refer to this as the tolerance effect. The repeated unnatural requests of a drug on our pleasure pathways wreck havoc with the system's feedback mechanisms. Maintaining artificially elevated levels of dopamine triggers the brain to decrease the sensitivity and number of dopamine receptors. In essence, your brain cells are being bludgeoned and become like the rock musician exposed to so much loud music he can only hear if you yell. That's why drug users—and, to a lesser extent, the pleasure seeker—need to keep upping their dose just to get the same lift. Eventually for drug addicts, the high is minimal, but they need the drug just to feel "normal."

It's easy to see the tolerance effect at work for power brokers, extreme skiers, and the rich and famous who can never get enough. But we can also observe this in ourselves, by noticing how we become bored with what we have and then quickly want better. As science journalist Robert Wright wrote, "Habituation to any goal—sex or power, say—is literally an addictive process, a growing dependence on the biological chemicals that make these things gratifying. The more power you have, the more you need. And any slippage will make you feel bad, even if it leaves you at a level that once brought ecstasy." Statistics show we have more than twice as many possessions as we did in 1960, yet we now work longer and spend more time shopping than ever. (Americans now spend more time shopping than the Russians did during the infamous long-line eras in the seventies and eighties.)

Our incessant busyness creates an anxiety and stress that we also get addicted to. Here, too, opioids play a role. If we remember that our stress response evolved for coping with and avoiding danger, such as escaping a bear, we see why painkillers and adrenaline get released when we're in trouble. So even if we're just worried about not making our deadline, our body/mind responds to that anxiety and panic as though we were physically threatened. Repeat that response again and again, and without being aware of it, we can get hooked on the endorphins that kick in during stress.

Opioids actually have a greater impact when we're under stress. This connection was first made during World War II when doctors noticed that soldiers badly wounded at the front needed much less or sometimes no morphine for injuries that civilians would have been agonized by. The extreme stress the soldiers had been under made their own endorphins extraordinarily potent. Clearly this is useful in battle situations, but when we regularly activate our stress response, over time it makes us more vulnerable to illness and depression.

How can we break these cycles?

LESSONS FROM TREATING ADDICTION

Obviously, we can't get rid of pleasure or the neurochemicals associated with it. Nor would we want to—even if we were a monk or nun meditating in a cave. Pleasure, like pain, can give us valuable information; it can indicate we're doing something right and help us remember what that is. The problem isn't pleasure itself, but becoming entranced with pleasure and making it our goal.

Lots of research has been done on the biochemistry of addiction. While all roads lead to the dopamine network, no one has been able to come up with a pill or shot that can eliminate an addiction. That's because addiction is really caused—or broken—by an intangible: motivation. This makes sense physiologically if you recall that a) our pleasure pathway is located in brain parts associated with both judgment and emotion, and b) it also plays an important role in learning. Motivation is the common link between judgment and emotion. And when our motivations are healthy, we end up learning things, and when they're askew, we often fall into addiction.

Behavioral research on addiction confirms the crucial role motivation plays in forming and breaking addiction. Tests done on mice find that they only become addicted to morphine-laced water if they've done it by choice. Similarly, statistics on patients who take painkillers for injury or illness show that they rarely turn into morphine addicts, even if they become physically addicted to the drug. Contrast that with someone who takes heroin to feel high and we understand that regardless of the drug treatment or recovery program, you need a strong will to break the habit.

Q

THE BEST INTENTIONS

While the connection between motivation and addiction is well known, few apply the implications of this beyond breaking addictions. Yet this research hints at an outlook to pleasure that's helpful for everyone: the quality and healthiness of our pleasures depends on the intentions connected to them. If we do something purely for pleasure's sake—whether bingeing on chocolate or trying to get rich—it's likely to lead to addiction problems and pain, pleasure's shadow. Compare that to visiting a sick person in the hospital. We feel good about that, and that pleasure won't leave us feeling disappointed or empty after it's gone.

Obviously, I've used simple examples. Our motivations are often complicated—a mixture of pure and selfish aims. Yet the point remains that the quality of our pleasure, and its after-taste, are colored by the intention behind the action.

After recognizing this, one could potentially start some heavy moralizing about good and bad behaviors. But it's important to remember that we're talking about biology. We're not following directives because a religious tradition says we should, but heeding the logic of healthy and unhealthy behaviors based on lots of rigorous research. This changes the meaning and flavor of good and bad actions, both in how we apply it to ourselves and how we judge others. When we realize we're doing something because we're following a natural order, doing so should be compelling without being oppressive. It's something like discovering that eating hydrogenated oil causes cancer and heart disease. Knowing this, common sense tells you to avoid it, but you wouldn't make others follow your diet; doing so would be to mix nutritional facts with moralism, creating a food fundamentalist.

The Buddha didn't teach about right and wrong, but skillful and unskillful actions. Unwholesome actions are underwritten by unhealthy motivations, leading them to hurt us and usually others. Not surprisingly, given our evolutionary-formed group social instincts, unskillful intentions tend to be those that wish others harm or are decidedly selfish. Regardless of whether this is divinely ordained, those instincts are so strong that even if we don't believe they apply to us, we still harm ourselves if we disregard them—creating stress and tension with each violation. Conversely, cultivating positive intentions, caring for and genuinely wanting the best for others, brings us happiness and a clear mind.

It's worth noting that even if our motivations are generally good, we can still get waylaid by the addictive aspects of a positive pursuit. As Karl Marx famously noted, religion can be an opiate. Of course, that applies to lots of other things too (including falling in love with your own economic theories). Still, it's important to recognize how even meditating can potentially have addictive aspects.

During a 10-day retreat, for example, if you've sat through a lot of pain, facing it squarely, but generally not resisting it, after a while, it's not uncommon to feel blissful. Since pain and pleasure go together, the bliss is a byproduct of processing pain—the fine residue of pleasure left from the mostly vaporized discomfort. Few complain about this side benefit, but it's easy to fall for these delightful feelings and crave them so that you're disappointed when they end. S.N. Goenka repeatedly warns against making these nice sensations the aim of one's meditation, yet many students get hooked on them anyway—at least for a while. They've taken the pleasure to be what they're ultimately looking for instead of seeing that it's a sign that they're on to something even better.

One way to check if one's meditation or spiritual practice is on track is by remembering the harmful aspects of an addiction. While doing something to the exclusion of other things is often a sign of obsession, it should be tested against a couple of key benchmarks: sensitivity and narcissism. Addictions tend to leave one insensitive, dulled, and habit-/self-centered. So if whatever you're doing is making you more sensitive in the best ways— more concerned for others, more aware, more intuitively wise— then bingo, it's something good, not a hallmark of addiction.

In some ways, meditating is like going through detox. Stripped of our usual diversions—television, books, e-mail, chitchat, wine—we're left with our fantasies and delusions. Over time, these too fall away. As we continually try to focus on the unadorned reality of the moment, little room is left for illusions. Despite our best intentions, though, losing our thought crutches is exceedingly difficult. At times we'll want to give up; other times we'll resent the treatment. Like the alcoholic or dope addict in detox, we may actually shake. But, as with completing a detox program, afterwards we feel more healthy and wholesome and, yes, sensitive. The currents of pleasure and pain which inevitably wash by us, appear as ephemeral currents, changing moments to be noticed, but not grasped after or scared by. We're riding the river toward freedom and peacefulness.

CHAPTER 14

THE NO-SELF STRATEGY

*Despite our every instinct to the contrary, there is one thing
that consciousness is not: some entity deep inside the brain
that corresponds to the "self," some kernel of awareness that
runs the show, as the "man behind the curtain" manipulated
the illusion of a powerful magician in* The Wizard of Oz.
*After more than a century of looking for it, brain researchers
have long since concluded that there is no conceivable place
for such a self to be located in the physical brain, and that
it simply doesn't exist.*

—Time *magazine*

The major "aha" insight that led to the Buddha's enlightenment, the key that freed him from his own suffering, was the realization that there is no self—no me, no my, no mine. He saw that we don't have an individual psyche or soul that migrates from lifetime to lifetime or rests in eternity as some ethereal representation of me-ness. "'I am' is a delusion," taught the Buddha. Once that delusion is gone, so is selfishness, grasping, attachment, and unhappiness.

But what did the Buddha mean by this? Aren't I here writing these words and you there reading them? If there is no self, who is having this experience? And who experiences the results of our actions or intentions?

These questions are difficult to answer because (in the vein of "are you still beating your wife?"), they contain an assumption: there must be a someone or some entity experiencing each moment. Yet, what we call "I" is actually an event; it's not a thing or a being, but a coming together of processes. These processes are subject to the laws of cause and effect, so that what is happening now does affect what comes later, but no single element or aspect of this stream is solid or unchanging.

If you recall from chapter 1, ideas define and object-ify; they give a sense of thingness when none is actually there (where is the water's essence when it turns to ice or steam?). So we run into problems when we try to pinpoint or nail down what is meant by a thingless interdependent process. By their very nature, these processes resist clear definition; our attempts to conceptualize them turn what is a multifaceted ungraspable happening—a non-thing—into a thing. It's as though we're trying to freeze a rainbow solid, trying to make something that is essentially temporal into something spatial. So when we hear classic Buddhist explanations to questions about self—there are "thoughts without a thinker," "feelings without a feeler," "experience without an experiencer"—they don't really make sense, unless we witness this ourselves.

It's important to remember that the Buddha's teaching of no-self was never intended as a doctrine to be believed in. It's not another idea to become attached to and defended, but a truth to realize. Of course it helps to have some understanding of what the Buddha meant by no-self, but such explanations aren't intended to be proofs. After all, how could you ever definitively establish the existence of a non-thing? Like parents who can't show their child a non-monster under the bed, the best you can do is show that you can't find it anywhere. Since our belief in a self is way stronger than a kid's fear of monsters, we can't expect that logic alone will evaporate our certainty. But at least if we intellectually get a sense that our self doesn't have the bedrock reality we normally assume, we can shift our orientation, and head in a less me-ful direction.

WHERE AM I?

Let's start by trying to find our self. We could be still and concentrate really hard or hunt about, using a mirror, photo albums, or witnesses. The only ground rule is that "you know what I mean" doesn't count. Look as hard as we want, though, and all we'll find are myriad changing feelings, ideas, images, memories, possessions, and sounds. But these details are artifacts; they aren't the self itself.

All the prime definitions for our "self" fail the test. We can't point to our name (hey, it could have been Chris Labowski or Randy Miller). We can't point to our body, or why would we say "my" body. We know that when we die, the corpse is no longer a self. We can't say it's our thoughts, since thoughts are so fleeting; we can't remember what we were thinking half an hour, let alone half a year, ago (researchers estimate that in the course of a day we have over 50,000 thoughts).

We can't say it's our memory, which has innumerable gaps (what, for example, were you doing on April 6, 1993). Also, even someone suffering from severe amnesia retains a sense of self. We can't even say it's our personality; otherwise what would it mean to have days when we're "not ourselves"? And which personality would it be—the you after your boss chewed you out, the one hanging out with good friends on a Saturday night, or the one on a blind date? Who we are is affected by the situation we're in. What would "you" be like if you lived in ancient Greece or 1740? Intuitively we recognize it's not meaningful to speak of a "me" outside of the context we are in and were formed by.

NO-THINGNESS

There is no self because no thing exists independently. To appreciate what is meant by this, let's first investigate the thingness of something simple like a loaf of bread. What could be a more obvious, everyday thing?

Like all so-called things, bread is made of other things. A basic bread is created from flour, water, yeast, and sugar. Take away the flour and you don't have bread; likewise leave out the water or yeast and the best you can hope for is matzoh. Bread's existence relies on many different ingredients and forces. Some conditions, such as heat for baking, are obvious, but there are countless other significant, but crucial conditions, like the proper amount of oxygen for rising or the right amount of moisture in the atmosphere (try baking bread underwater). Everyone understands this, but they don't necessarily realize that what we're *really* saying is that bread doesn't exist on its own; it's not an independent thing. As the coming together of various factors, it has no intrinsic "breadness" itself.

The examination of ingredients and necessary conditions for making bread could go on and on, revealing—depending upon how you look at it—either its interdependence with all things or a complete lack of independent, intrinsic breadness. Consider the heat for the baking. It probably comes from electricity and the electricity comes from a power plant which relies on coal. Coal production needs coal miners and equipment; the equipment was made in a factory and so forth. An investigation downward into the loaf's ingredients, what we might consider its essential building blocks, shows a dramatic lack of solidity.

Investigating flour, for instance, we find it is composed of wheat fibers. The wheat fibers in turn are really patterns of wheat cells. The wheat cells are composed of molecules; the molecules made of atoms, and the atoms created from patterns of subatomic particles. All these "entities," down to the very smallest, are made up of other things (indeed how could there even be a single smallest *thing*, as then that could be cut in half itself to create a still smaller thing?). And all these "things" are constantly changing. Looking at atoms and their subatomic parts—those entities which come closest to the title of "the basic building blocks of all things"—reveals truly awesome challenges to our notions of solidity and thingness.

Atoms are almost entirely empty space. What makes up an atom (to keep things simple) is a nucleus and teensy, weensy electrons. The weight of the nucleus accounts for 99.9 percent of an atom's mass, and this relatively powerful presence keeps the electrons in their orbit. Yet the nucleus is still actually very, very, very, very small compared to the whole space the atom takes up—which is of course incredibly tiny itself (about one hundred-millionth of a centimeter if that means anything to you; if it doesn't, consider that to see the atoms in an orange, you'd need to expand the fruit to be about the size of the earth). To get a sense of the incredible lack of solidity in an atom we need to do some more imaginary enlarging on a gigantic scale. Expand an atom to the size of a large room, for example, and you still wouldn't detect the nucleus. To see a nucleus the size of a grain of salt, we'd have to enlarge an atom to be as big as a fourteen-story building. Enlarge further, by making the nucleus the size of a softball, and the nearest orbiting electron, roughly the size of a piece of salt, would be about $\frac{1}{2}$ mile away.

But before getting comfortable with these visual analogies, note that it's largely misleading to even think of atoms and subatomic particles in spatial terms—as things. The movement of particles is so lightning fast, their existence so uncertain and ephemeral, so constantly changing—first assuming this form and then another—as to make it accurate to say they both exist and don't exist at the same time. As Gary Zukav put it in *The Dancing Wu Li Masters*, his bestselling book about physics:

> What we have been calling matter (particles) constantly is being created, annihilated and created again. This happens as particles interact and it also happens, literally, out of nowhere.

> Where here was "nothing" there suddenly is "something," and then the something is gone again, often changing into something else before vanishing. In particle physics there is no distinction between empty, as in "empty space," and not-empty, or between something and not-something. The world of particle physics is a world of sparkling energy forever dancing with itself in the form of its particles as they twinkle in and out of existence, collide, transmute, and disappear again.

We too are made up of vibrant peek-a-boo energy and we too are interconnected to the whole universe (try doing without oxygen, water, or microbes). Obviously our awareness makes us much different than a loaf of pumpernickel, yet the Buddha discovered that even our experience could be divided into major ingredients—the psychophysical equivalents of flour, water, sugar and yeast. The Buddha found every experience involves five rapidly changing interdependent processes, each arising attached to one of our six faculties (our five senses and the ability to think). His awareness was so refined, he was able to dissect how these constituents or aggregates, as he called them, worked together. Doing so, he scooped modern neuroscientists by about 2,600 years. As it's only recently that cognitive researchers are concluding that there is indeed no single agent or place inside us where cognition takes place.

Nowhere in our brain is there a definitive neuron or group of neurons that act like a small core being or true mini-me that needs to register an experience for it to count as an experience. Rather, research on cognition shows that the brain works through separate subsystems, each handling its own task, rather than going through a central headquarters which must be involved in all our experiences. Imaging technologies have shown just how specific these subsystems can be. The colors red and green, for instance, are handled by different spots in the visual cortex. As science philosopher Daniel Dennett wrote about trying to investigate *who* is actually seeing: "You enter the brain through the eye, march up the optic nerve, round and round the cortex, looking behind every neuron, and then before you know it, you emerge into daylight on the spike of a motor nerve impulse, scratching your head and wondering where the self is."

While few humans have the awareness prowess to witness the rapid, subconcious details of their cognitive processes, without any training we can detect the absence of a single operator controlling the show. Try this simple, if subtle exercise: look at something intently and then switch your attention to listening. Then stare at the first thing again. Now see if you can both see and hear at the same time. If you really focus, you'll notice that you switch back and forth very quickly between the two. It seems like we experience many of our senses at once, but really this is just a false impression that comes from the speed of our cognitive processes. Consciousness is actually discontinuous.

As long as we continue to believe that the looking, listening, and switching are being done by the same self, by me, then this exercise is unlikely to impress you. But what would it mean to be the same entity when different bodily parts and mechanisms and different objects—things which aren't even inside our body—"create" the experiences? If, for example, you heard wind rustling leaves, where did that sound happen? Is it where the air passed through the branches? In your eardrum? Or in the part of your brain that processes soft sounds? The more one thinks about it, the more the experience seems not like something we are doing, but as an event that happened. There was no one in charge of it, just as there is no one in charge of making a tree grow or the wind blow. Even the exercise we just did wasn't your idea or even my idea. (I got it from Wes Nisker's book *Buddha's Nature*; who knows where he got it from?)

Once we truly realize that we are not an objective unmoved observer, separate from what is now unfolding, we can live the truth of selflessness. When that happens the anxiety and numbness we feel from trying to run and hold ourselves apart from this moment stops. As it turns out, our usual idea of ultimate freedom—to be able to remove ourselves from any situation—is not only a fantasy, it's exactly the opposite of what real freedom is: having no resistance to whatever is.

UNDERSTANDING OUR SENSE(S) OF SELF

If you're stubborn or terribly clever, maybe you could construct some metaphysical or conceptual model of the self—say Kant's transcendental ego-self—that tries to account for how a self could experience constant change, be different every moment, and yet still remain the same thing. But, as cognitive scientist Francisco Varela noted in *The Embodied Mind*, this theoretical soul still wouldn't really work as an explanation since that isn't what we mean by our sense of self. The feeling of "me" is immediate, visceral, and real. It's not something we need to ponder to create.

So where does this instinctive sense of self come from? Most likely it's yet another evolutionary adaptation. Daniel Dennett points out that, at the simplest level, self-awareness lets an organism know some basic, but important information such as "When hungry, don't eat yourself!" and "When there's pain, it's yours!" No doubt all animals must have at least some rudimentary sense of this to function.

Self-awareness also seems necessary for organizing and prioritizing our actions. Like the old Yiddish expression says: "You can't dance at two weddings with only one tush." Since we can only do one thing at a time, we need a mechanism for deciding what we should do, and for coordinating the various body parts needed to actually pull it off. Otherwise the whole organism wouldn't survive. If being hungry, for example, didn't grab "our" attention over say sniffing a rose, we wouldn't last very long. This is probably why we are so identified with our will; by identifying with actions we need to take, we can complete tasks.*

Note, however, the difference between a basic, functional sense of self and having an ego. An ego seems to be an adaptation designed for competitive social situations. It helps us keep score in the tit-for-tat game which characterizes many of our exchanges ("Look at all I've done for him!"). Maintaining an estimate of our skills, prowess, and reputation helps us figure out how much we can get away with and get for ourselves. Tracking other selves lets

---

* Two points to note for this paragraph and the one above:

• Speaking of a "whole organism" is a convenience, like using the terms "I," "me," "you," etc. Remember that an "individual" is made of processes, not to mention a conglomeration of other countless smaller organisms—all crucial to each other's survival. After remarking that most creatures exist as a collective of many organisms, zoologist Matt Ridley wrote, "What is an organism? There is no such thing."

• Lest we start thinking our will or intention to carry out actions is the real "me" or "I" we're looking for, note that our will also works through impersonal mechanisms. In *How the Mind Works*, Steven Pinker writes that "the agents of the brain might very well be organized hierarchically into nested subroutines with a set of master decision rules, a computational demon or agent . . . , sitting at the top of the chain of command. It would not be a ghost in the machine, just another set of if-then rules or a neural network that shunts control to the loudest, fastest, or strongest agent one level down." Such a set up doesn't eliminate free will, it just limits it to responses to our present situation.

us know who we can trust and who we should fear. The more formidable, wonderful, or important we seem, the more likely it is that others will help or respect us. While this makes practical, if crude, sense, why should we be taken in by our own self-puffery? For the same reason (as noted in chapter 10) that we fall for our other self-deceptions: it makes them more convincing. It's hard to persuade others of our greatness, strength, kindness, innocence, or claims of self-sacrifice without believing it ourselves.

So what does having two different senses of self—one functional and one ego-centered—suggest? First, that losing our ego doesn't imply self-annihilation or suicide. One can stop identifying with our experiences as something we own and "me" as a thing, and still function perfectly well. We needn't worry that losing our ego will turn us into a blob, unable to feed and clothe ourselves and liable to walk into moving traffic.

Second, since our sense of self is a very powerful instinct, if we wish to see through the illusion of me, my, and mine, we must be patient and skillful. There's no point to bullying ourselves out of having a sense of self. In the Pali Canon, there is a story of a nearly enlightened monk named Khemaka who had clearly witnessed the five aggregates operating; he realizes without any doubt that there is truly no separate self. Yet, he admits to still having the vague feeling "I am." Although Khemaka eventually loses even this whiff of self, if such an advanced monk retains this feeling, there is no reason to pretend we have lost it when we haven't.

A sense of self can't be beaten out of us through self-flogging, sermons, or asceticism. As long as we have a sense of me, we should treat ourselves and other selves kindly. This doesn't suggest self-indulgence or self-aggrandizement, but love, respect, and tolerance. Once a selfless awareness is a living reality, abundant compassion will flow naturally—in the same way we don't need to convince our right hand to be nice to our left.

Third, it's largely our ego that creates problems for us. The less ego-based we are, the more peaceful we'll be. Egotism is the root of selfishness and the nature of selfishness is grabbiness: wanting more, more, more for ME. So freedom from selfishness is freedom from wanting—the cause of our discontent.

Nearly everything in the Buddha's Eight-fold Path undermines egotism in some way. Maintaining the precepts brings a certain baseline of humility, keeps us from outright selfishness, and reminds us of the other guy. And meditation can help us actually observe that what we mistake for our self is only made of fleeting processes. Meditation also helps to diffuse egotism both by providing a break from the social pressures that tend to breed ego building and by getting us to concentrate on something beside ourselves. After meditating for a while, we're struck by how much time and energy normally goes toward spiffing up our egos. At some point, most meditators realize, "My god, I am an egomaniac."

Given that the ego's main role is a competitive one, it makes sense that reducing its hold on us would feel healing. Competing is stressful. Even if you're good at it or find moments of calm during competition, it doesn't nourish peacefulness. Think of the people you know who are ruthlessly competitive and invariably you'll find big egos. Likewise, most serious egotists are very competitive. For blatant examples, think of dictators who will do anything to stay on top or boxers who build themselves up so they can pummel opponents. No matter how successful they are, these can't be genuinely content people.*

The lesson to take from this isn't that we should be meek, self-effacing, or falsely modest. Of course given our tendency to over-inflate (or deflate) our own image, adding a few dollops of moderation to our self-assessments tends to keep us more truth-

---

* Note the difference, when top athletes, even boxers, attribute their success to god or some spiritual force; not only are they better sportsman, but also have happier, better lives outside the sporting arena.

ful, but how we come off is irrelevant. It's honesty and freedom from needing to build up our ego that we're after. Genuinely owning up to mistakes and flaws feels liberating because we can let go of pretending to be a somebody or a something we're not. Any role we identify with creates a certain amount of stress. The freedom we feel when we take a break from fueling or attaching to our egos hints at the bliss we'd feel if we totally dropped all our identities.

SIDE-STEPPING SELF-WORTH: THE NO-SELF STRATEGY

Our culture tends to be mystified or even hostile to the idea of egolessness. We've been taught that the secret to happiness is to feel good about ourselves. While there's some truth in that (certainly genuine compassion begins at home), cultivating egotism is not an effective antidote to a poor self-image. It only covers over the real issues one must face.

Conventional wisdom has it that violent crimes are committed largely by people with low self-esteem, but recent research indicates the opposite: violent crimes may be committed by those with excessive, untenably *high* self-esteem. What many criminals and violent political leaders, such as Hitler, Stalin, or Saddam Hussein, have in common is excessive narcissism—a self-regard that turns violent when threatened.

Roy F. Baumeister, a Case Western Reserve psychologist, who has extensively studied violence, wrote in *Scientific American*: "There is nothing wrong with helping [children] . . . and others take pride in accomplishments and good deeds, but there is plenty of reason to worry about encouraging people to think highly of themselves when they haven't earned it. Conceited, self-important individuals turn nasty toward those who puncture their bubbles of self-love." Karen Armstrong, a scholar of Western religions, has observed that essentially says the same thing: "Egotism can arguably be described as the source of all evil."

At the moment, our concern isn't with what causes violence and no doubt it's not solely the result of an overblown self-image (we've all met serious narcissists who are gentle enough). Rather, the point is to see how building up egos isn't a sound corrective for low self-esteem or a good tactic for real contentment. Exceedingly low and excessively high self-esteem actually seem to be flip sides of the same problem: a lack of acceptance of our experiences. Unable to tolerate what they feel, the person with low self-esteem turns violent against themselves, those with high self-regard rage against others.

Acceptance, coupled with awareness and wisdom, is what can release us from a domineering sense of self—whether our ego is browbeating or seducing us. By focusing on our moment-to-moment feelings, actions, and intentions, we can attend to our acceptance of this moment (which is essentially created by our past actions and intentions) while creating a genuinely positive future.

We usually think that our psychological problems come from some *thing* inside us that needs fixing, as if a good personality surgeon could repair it. So when the problem crops up again and again, we feel defeated by it; it seems as if there is little we can do to rid ourselves of the burdens we're stuck with. But when we remember "we" are only composed of processes, we realize what we really have is a cause-and-effect problem. This can only be changed by changing how we react in the moment, not just by thinking of ourselves differently or even *only* by insight into our past traumas.

Both positive and negative states of mind aren't static, but need feeding to live. So, for example, if we feel stingy while giving someone an obligatory gift, we might contract and complain, telling ourselves the person we're giving to has never gotten us anything good; essentially, this strengthens that feeling of stinginess and makes it more likely to arise again. If instead, we could stay aware of the tightness we feel, without denying or trying to change it, it will eventually disappear. We can also consciously cultivate feelings of generosity and good wishes toward the person we're giving to (knowing we're the one who really gets hurt by our miserliness). This weakens the feeling further and plants a positive state of mind. As the Buddha said, "Our life is shaped by our mind. We become what we think. Suffering follows an evil thought as the wheels of a cart follow the oxen that draw it." Naturally, the reverse is also true: "Joy follows a pure thought like a shadow that never leaves."

By tending to our issues in the present, we largely bypass questions about what sort of person we are. This may sound strange at first: how will I become a good person, if I don't worry about it? But fretting over whether I'm kind, accomplished, or worthy generally isn't productive. Judging ourselves only tends to puncture or pump up our ego, setting ourselves up for more disappointment and denial when we do make mistakes—all the while taking our eye off the ball of what is happening right now.

When we do need to review something we've done, a better strategy is to concentrate on our actions, noting whether we've handled things well and whether we can learn something from it. Essentially this is what enlightened parenting guides now tell us; they advise that we compliment our children with "good job" instead of "good boy." We can do the same thing for ourselves. When we realize we've made a mistake, it's better to focus on what we need to do better next time and the resolve to do it rather than wallow in guilt, which only tends to sap our energy.

We can use this basic approach for incorporating any insightful analysis we have into our patterns—whether that insight came from our own introspection or from something a friend, therapist, or partner has told us. Knowing our trouble spots, we should try to be even more sensitively aware in those situations, but, ideally, without becoming overly identified with the problem. Recognizing, for example, that we were victimized as a child is very informative, but becoming a victim is debilitating. No matter how much work you do around understanding the event(s) of your abuse, you'll still have to work skillfully with the way that wound manifests itself in the present. So if we tend to beat ourselves up, try to be aware of that pattern as it happens without supporting it and giving it sustenance. Over time the impulse for self-recrimination will weaken. The real art is in being aware of negative or harmful impulses without either giving in to them *or* squashing them.

Ironically, by concentrating on what we're doing and feeling—instead of on who we are—we end up being more like the person we hope to be. It's a lesson we've all learned before, but tend to forget time and again: by focusing on process instead of results, we actually end up with better results. To paraphrase the monk and teacher Thanissaro Bhikkhu, by staying aware of how we handle our present feelings and intentions, we can master the processes of cause and effect that shape our life. This is how every great artist or craftsman develops mastery and skill.

CHAPTER 15

WHAT ABOUT NIRVANA?

No Buddhist idea has proved as problematic for the European mind as that of Nirvana.
　　—*Stephen Batchelor,*
　　The Awakening of the West: The Encounter of
　　Buddhism and Western Culture

What *did* the Buddha experience when he became enlightened? This question, which is basically the same as asking "what is nirvana?" has long been a magnet for speculation—and understandably so. Those who experience nirvana, even for a few moments, speak of an inconceivable peacefulness, a boundless tranquility that evaporates confusion. For most Buddhists, this realization is the goal of their spiritual efforts. And even those who don't set their sights on enlightenment come to see that the Buddha's own awakening, his clear experience of nirvana, is the source for what he taught. This doesn't imply that you must make enlightenment your aim to benefit from meditation or the Buddha's path; yet if Siddhartha Gautama hadn't realized this final truth, this ultimate erasing of boundaries and suffering, he would not have had a new perspective to impart, no Noble Truths to expound, no new way to pass along—essentially no Buddhism.

While it's natural to want to know what nirvana is like, this yearning has led to many misconceptions, misunderstandings which apparently were also common during the Buddha's lifetime. After hearing about nirvana, for example, most of us tend to think of it as a place or a state of mind, a sort of exceptionally pleasant and calm holding pattern. Even if we picture it in a very vague and ephemeral way, no matter how sketchy, intense, or exaggerated we imagine it to be, we end up with some version of an experience that's at least something like what we already know. Conversely, others imagine that nirvana is the annihilation of all experience, the kind of nothingness that most atheists imagine when they think of death. According to the Buddha, this thought is actually a projection; a scenario that scares us when we crave eternal life and comforts us when we desire an escape from life's trials. Evidently none of the above assumptions about nirvana is true.

While it's relatively easy to say what nirvana is not, it's essentially impossible to say what it is. This is because nirvana is beyond the realm of normal perception. One can make vague, incomplete attempts to describe it, but about the only definitive, non-negative characteristic you can ascribe to nirvana is that it's Ultimate Reality—Truth with a forever capital "T." Beyond that, even those who are intimately familiar with nirvana must describe it in negative terms. Here's what the Buddha is reported to have said about it:

> There is a sphere of experience that is beyond the
> entire field of matter, the entire field of mind, that is

neither this world nor another world nor both, neither moon nor sun. This I call neither arising, nor passing away, nor abiding, neither dying nor rebirth. It is without support, without development, without foundation. This is the end of suffering.

...

There is an unborn, unbecome, uncreated, unconditioned. Were there not an unborn, unbecome, uncreated, unconditioned, no release would be known from the born, the become, the created, the conditioned.

...

Here the four elements of solidity, fluidity, heat and motion have no place; the notions of length and breadth, the subtle and the gross, good and evil, name and form are altogether destroyed; neither this world nor the other, nor coming, going, or standing, neither death nor birth, nor sense-objects are to be found.

What does it mean to be beyond the field of mind and matter and all notions of relativity or comparison? The short answer, and the only truly reliable one, is that we can't know unless we experience it. And since you can only experience nirvana by being totally aligned with just what is, trying to imagine nirvana only makes its realization more unlikely—and impossible in that moment of imagination.

We don't have to assume, however, that the nirvanic case is closed and that all efforts to make sense of enlightenment must end. The nirvanic experience can be framed in nonmystical terms that improves one's appreciation and practice of Buddhism. If this weren't possible, it seems all died-in-the-wool rationalists would have to stop right here. For how could they accept a "you'll see when you get there" answer when "there" sounds so fuzzy?

The rationale underlying a practical understanding of nirvana has two aspects: first, we must let go of what we can't logically know—such as what nirvana is like, "who" experiences it, or is it eternal after death? Second, we must focus on what we can possibly understand by building on what has conclusively been said about it. By letting go of trying to rationally comprehend *the experience* of nirvana, we're not signing off on using rationality, we're simply recognizing its limits. In Intro to Philosophy one is asked to consider whether an all-powerful God could make a round square (or was it a square circle?). Trying to answer this feels, at best, more like entertainment than the pursuit of wisdom: we know we can't really learn anything significant from it. Similarly, if experiencing nirvana means to go beyond mind and matter, to apprehend what could be called another dimension, then, by definition, trying to portray that experience in our familiar three-dimensional terms would be impossible. This doesn't imply that this other dimension is elsewhere, just that it can't translate into our usual forms in a comprehensible way. Most animals, for example, have a sense of space without a sense of time. This doesn't mean time refers to another place or plane (at least not in a spatial way).

So let's review the few things that have definitively been said about nirvana. Foremost, is that it is Ultimate Truth, unconditioned Reality, unadorned "as isness." Second, as already stressed, apprehending this ultimate Wisdom is beyond our normal channels of perception. Last, should one experience this Truth, it has a purifying effect. Even a fleeting experience of it dispels anxiety, craving, and selfishness. Becoming drenched in it brings a lasting, unshakeable contentment. While these claims may initially sound grand, they can at least be considered.

Many of us bristle at the very the idea of Absolute Truth. But when we look closer at that irritation, we usually find it's not the idea of truth that's bothersome, but the resulting violence or oppression that ensues after one makes claims of exclusivity or restricted access. It's true that the Buddha realized something others hadn't so in that sense his realization was exclusive—or, to be more accurate, rarified—but he maintained it is available to anyone. Furthermore, he devoted his life to showing others how to have this insight.

Since the Buddha never ascribed any graspable qualities to nirvana, there's really no details to fight over or defend. When asked, for example, whether God existed or not, the Buddha maintained a "noble silence" knowing that answering either way would be misleading and problematic. So without particular qualities ascribed to the Truth, one can't really quibble with the report; you can only object to either the idea that Truth could exist or, even if it did, that it could be recognized. This objection is a familiar modern belief, one that seems necessary to hold in a pluralistic society, but it's actually self-contradictory: to say that the truth can't be known, is to state a different truth.

Most of us have a deep sense that some kind of truth exists and that it matters, even if we're only prepared to accept a slippery, moment-to-moment authenticity. Certainly the pursuit of truth is the source of all scientific understanding and indeed any legitimate knowledge we do have. Still, it seems that if science has shown anything, it's that our knowledge is forever being revised and refined. In that context, how can we make sense of the Buddha's claim to Absolute Truth? One way is to consider how he may have gone beyond the reaches of science. Science, after all, studies the measurable. Yet this is exactly what the Buddha did not experience. As unfamiliar as that may sound, many scientists know enough to see science's limits and have concluded that it's logical to assume there is some reality beyond what we can normally apprehend.

SOME HINTS FROM SCIENCE'S FRONTIERS

Einstein's most famous scientific insights suggest that our usual understanding of reality is limited and misleading. His special theory of relativity works based on the assumption that space and time are inseparable from each other and reality itself. This idea overturns our intuitive, Newtonian sense that things happen spatially in three-dimensions, distinct from time which is absolute and marches forward independently of what takes place. Not so, says Einstein, since a sequence of events are relative to an observer's position and velocity, the "same" event can occur at different times for different observers. So if multiple, indeed infinite, scenarios for the "same" event are possible, how could one be an independent "true" time? Why would any single observer's vantage point be the real, accurate one? Whatever is, is—now; reality can't in fact be separated into a before, now, and then, even if that's how we experience it. Countless experiments by physicists indicate that reality is actually four-dimensional (that is, time is inseparable from things/events). So based on Einstein's theory of relativity, physicists conclude that it's more accurate to think of space and time as not moving. "Events do not develop, they just are," explains Gary Zukav in *The Dancing Wu Li Masters*, his award-winning book on physics. To complete that idea, Zukav explains:

> If we could view our reality in a four-dimensional way, we would see that everything that now seems to unfold before us with the passing of time, already exits in toto, painted as it were, on the fabric of space-time. We would see all, the past, the present, and the future with one glance. . . .

> Don't worry about visualizing a four-dimensional world. Physicists can't do it, either.

This sense of experiencing all and nothing at the same time is a consistent insight from those who've had a genuinely transcendent experience.

Though we're sure we see reality accurately, what we really experience are creations, or partial creations, of "our" mind. Neuroscientists have concluded that our nervous system detects less than one part per billion of the total energy vibrating in the environment. As Sir John Eccles, an eminent British neurologist explained, "realize that there is no color in the natural world and no sound—nothing of this kind; no textures, no patterns, no beauty, no scent." In other words, hearing or seeing something depends upon, and is shaped by, our senses and nervous system. There is, for instance, no actual redness in the universe or in an object itself. Red appears when photons hit the rods and cones in our retina, etc., in a certain way. The red we experience is *subjectively* accurate or "true," it just doesn't have an absolute grounding. "Things" don't have a reality independent of the experience and mind that give it substance (and vice versa).

Even when we experience something based on external information, it is still a mental construct, explains New York University Medical School neuroscientist Dr. Rodolfo Llinas. As Llinas put it, "Is there a sound if a tree drops in the forest and no one hears it? No. Sound is the relationship between external vibrations and the brain. If there is no brain, there can be no sound." The upshot, according to Llinas: "We can say that being awake or being conscious is nothing but a dreamlike state." Even if, he adds, this state corresponds closely to some "external" reality and others can collaborate the experience, it has no objective reality—it's like a rainbow.

Such science can make our heads spin because our sense of reality and Reality is shaped by our boundaries, by how we take it all in. It's very difficult to accept that everything we experience—our fundamental base for everything we believe in—is not objectively, inherently real or strictly accurate.

Consider, though, what would happen if we had an experience beyond our familiar ones, in which time and space were not separate. Imagine *the effect* of experiencing existence without even a trace of interpretation. It makes no sense to imagine what the experience itself would be like because it would be unlike anything we've ever known. Remember, it is "beyond mind and matter," beyond our usual channels of perception. But we can easily understand that if we did have this experience, it would clear up a great deal of confusion. And that afterwards, we'd be enlightened to at least some extent.

WHAT TO MAKE OF ALL THIS

After considering the possibility of experiencing Reality truly as it is, without filters, beyond mind and matter, you're likely to veer toward one of two opposite reactions: either you'll be skeptical that anyone could have such an encounter or balk at how unspiritual it sounds. For those who dislike the clinical ring, note that experiencing nirvana isn't something that can be willed to happen or found through technical means. To experience reality as-it-is, one must be totally open, unblocked, and in touch with what is. This requires a great deal of what could be called spiritual or psychological work. To develop to such a point, one needs to have weakened the shields—our egotism, craving, fear, and attachments—which both freeze our heart and prevent us from seeing things as they are. It's said that to be ripe for nirvana one must develop the following ten qualities: generosity, morality, renunciation, wisdom, effort, tolerance, truth, determination, selfless love, and equanimity. Knowing this, we can see how most religions, therapies, and efforts to be a better person move us in some way toward wisdom. The Ultimate Truth the Buddha and others have experienced shouldn't be thought of as truth in a narrow, factual sense, but more as Ultimate Wisdom.

According to this tradition of vipassana, anyone who's had even an instant of witnessing Absolute Truth—a nirvanic dip as they say—experiences a kind of cleansing that dispels existential illusions. With greater and extended awakenings, one also finds one has a basic moral purity which makes it unlikely one will act in a grossly unethical way again. This doesn't imply that after experiencing nirvana all one's troubles or egotism vanish, but a certain baseline wisdom and kindness will follow.

If we haven't experienced this ourselves, it's understandable to be at least a little skeptical. Even accepting that one can experience nirvana requires some faith. Those who commit themselves to this practice, tend to find that faith grows because what they've already learned to be true for themselves is consistent with what's ahead. We may never fully realize or even get a glimpse of Ultimate Truth ourselves, but by living truthfully, with wisdom, we can experience a watered-down, but still palpable liberation and peacefulness that gives benefits here and now. I once asked vipassana teacher and psychotherapist Paul Fleischman, "How do we know it's truly possible to experience nirvana?" He answered, "The Buddha may have been the greatest con man who ever lived, but even if he was, I still find this practice leads to a good life, one I'd choose again and again." Obviously Fleischman wasn't suggesting the Buddha was lying, but that he's gotten enough from doing this practice that it doesn't really matter whether it's possible for him to experience nirvana himself.

To evaluate whether this path, or any direction we're heading in, is worthwhile, it seems wise to consider any underlying principle(s) informing that direction. In this light, nirvana can be understood as the end point along a continuum we can all experience as we move toward greater truthfulness and wisdom. We may never get to that end point, but we can tell if heading that way is a good thing.

Everything in the Buddha's path—from moral precepts, which help keep us honest, to meditation, which directs us to witness what is as objectively as possible—aligns us with truth. If nirvana is Absolute Truth, truth in its purest form, to be able to realize it, we must embody truth, honesty, and wisdom as much as possible in our life. Knowing this, we realize that ultimate wisdom can't be found through a mechanical formula; it becomes clear why we're told that you can meditate until your bones become brittle, but if you haven't developed your overall purity, you'll never become enlightened.

By regarding the Buddha's path as a dedication to truth, wisdom, and losing our protective shields, it's easy to see how it's compatible with other religions and complemented by any solid humanist value such as generosity, tolerance, courage, kindness, etc. There's no reason one couldn't be a dedicated atheist or devoted Catholic, Jew, Hindu, etc., and still follow the Buddha's prescription. Even if your cosmology doesn't agree with what the Buddha found, you could still use his methods as a tool. For the essential point is to develop wisdom, bathed in truthfulness.

When we embrace honesty, we find clarity mixed with uncertainty. Along with a greater calm and softness, we find our own violence, anger, struggle, and ignorance—making it harder to be judgmental of "sinners." We see that even as we're getting wiser, we're still mostly confused. Oddly, though, one's faith isn't really shaken by this uncertainty. Instead, we see the futility of grasping and trying to understand everything; beliefs appear more like guiding lights than walls which lock us inside. Wall-less, we find more freedom than we ever knew was possible.

As we all know from our finer moments, honesty feels liberating. Or as Jesus said (and he wasn't just referring to his own words, but to "the Spirit of truth"), "the truth will set you free." It seems this is so every step of the way—up to the very last one.

CHAPTER 16

CONCLUSION:

ON EFFORT, DOUBT, AND ENLIGHTMENT

Suppose a man were wounded by an arrow smeared with poison, and brought to a surgeon. The man would say: "I will not let the surgeon pull out the arrow until I know the name and clan of the man who wounded me; whether the bow that wounded me was a long bow or a crossbow; whether the arrow that wounded me was hoof-tipped or curved or barbed."

All this would still not be known to that man and meanwhile he would die. So too, if anyone should say: "I will not lead the noble life under the Buddha until the Buddha declares to me whether the world is eternal or not eternal, finite or infinite; whether the soul is the same as or different from the body; whether or not an awakened one continues or ceases after death," that would still remain undeclared by the Buddha and meanwhile that person would die.

—The Buddha

The Buddha's last words, uttered just before he died, urged his followers to work diligently for their freedom. The aim: complete enlightenment, the cessation of suffering, the end of defilements, and union with the unborn. Though people are drawn to meditate for different reasons, ultimately this is what most Buddhists are after.

Yet, using even the most optimistic and generous accounting, fully enlightened people are very rare. In *After the Ecstasy, the Laundry,* insight meditation teacher Jack Kornfield highlights this by recounting stories of teachers who still have problems. These advanced students and meditation masters have experienced great spiritual heights, they embody a tremendous source of wisdom, and live mostly peaceful, inspiring lives—at least for long stretches. But Kornfield (who is no spiritual slouch himself) has yet to meet anyone who is immune from unhappiness or psychic discomfort. In Tibet, a land known for enlightened beings and big mountains, there's an expression: "Your guru should live three valleys away." It's likely the Dalai Lama would agree, or at least smile, since he doesn't claim to be a perfected human himself. Neither, for that matter, does S.N. Goenka.

So what are us more ordinary folks to do? Is there any point to our efforts?

In one's lesser moments, it's easy to be cynical about the mote in our guru's eyes. "See, they're just like us," we scoff and sigh, relieved we're not the only ones who screw up, yet disappointed we don't have unblemished heroes. But this response doesn't leave us much to go on. Recognizing we're all human is important; it suggests we should avoid self-proclaimed sages, who act like mean-spirited fools, or worse. Yet, it's also important not to let a naive idealism distract us from seeing, and working with, what is. Facing flaws shouldn't turn into a justification not to make an effort. "If *they* aren't saints, how can I be expected to be?" can easily turn into spiritual whining.

Such complaints are understandable of course, but soon enough, whether we consciously think it through or not, we're likely to recognize that even if perfection is beyond me, even if it's beyond everyone I know, I must do what those who are truly wiser than me have done, and continue to do: keep moving forward with as much honesty and good judgment as possible. The Buddha never claimed his path was easy. He offered no package deals for a quick nirvana or short cuts to a pleasant afterlife. He gave us an authentic, practical plan, but it's a workfare program. And a hard one at that.

Expecting quick results is a kind of immaturity. The hope for an easy release denies the real work we have to do. Nonetheless, most of us, at least sometimes, lean in this direction. When that happens, it's worth remembering the importance of patience and forbearance, the foot soldiers of any campaign to change. Naturally this doesn't suggest we should only trudge straight ahead, allowing ourselves to be infiltrated by complacency, the "near-enemy" of patience or stiffness, the gone-wrong cousin of forbearance. We should be aware if we're making some sort of progress, but without big expectations. In other words, a realistic yet light touch is in order.

Trust and willpower are opposite faculties which must be harmoniously balanced and accompanied by wisdom for our efforts to be effective and satisfying. We've all met people who rely too much on either willpower or trust, resulting in control freaks or daydreamers. But with the right mix of faith, determination, and wisdom, we can cut a swath through uncertainty, difficulties, and mixed emotions. Determination gives us energy, faith keeps us moving forward, and wisdom provides the aim. And all the while, it's good to remember the Buddha's First Noble Truth: that life is inherently dissatisfying. We should *expect* that the road ahead will be bumpy, slippery, or in some way not just as we want it. No method or approach to life will seem perfect and unambiguously right for us. Why should a spiritual path be different from everything else?

If it sounds like I'm giving a bit a pep talk to myself as well as you, you're right. Although as I write these words my confidence in the Buddha's way is very strong, odds are that at some point I'll have moments of doubt. When considered in retrospect, that doubt doesn't reflect a mistake in the Buddha's teaching, but mirrors my own frustrations, typically a case of expectations leading to desire. Still, after watching an unflattering self-portrait in the mirror of recall, I sometimes wonder if I'm really making progress or just struggling in quicksand?

This is a good question. Pretending to be someone we're not, or know something we don't, doesn't do anyone any good. Doubt isn't something to fear. It's important to recognize and even honor uncertainty. It keeps us from reaching for easy answers and from using our beliefs for security. The positive aspect of doubt is that it can also loosen our grip on any ideologies or opinions we're clinging to.

But of course doubt can also have a debilitating effect. So after honestly facing it, we must eventually do something. After disappointment and the questions left in its wake pass, I do what all of us must, no matter what path we follow (or don't): I pick myself up, dust myself off, and try to do better for the umpteen millionth time. Until we're without flaws, or we drop, it's all we can ever do.

Some Buddhists, conceding enlightenment in their lifetime is unlikely, see this as a long-term project. Their efforts are partially fueled by expectations of rebirth. They very well may be right; in fact, if I *had to* bet, I'd put my chips with them. But even if this go-round is all we've got and we fall far short of enlightenment, following the Buddha's prescription still has much to offer. Even if we never become fully aware, boundlessly compassionate, or flawlessly ethical, by putting our efforts in that direction, by heading toward the light, we're still more likely to embody those qualities, making us—at the very least—somewhat happier and somewhat lighter as we go. And since everyone needs to pick themselves up countless times, how nice to be carrying less weight. So many people, through blindness and misbehavin', seem to pile on troubles. As they advance in years, not only must they contend with flagging energy and aching bones, but growing burdens—the legacy of bad intentions and poor choices.

Near the end of the Buddha's life, when it was obvious that within a few months he too would go the way of all compounded things, the Buddha's attendant, Ananda, asked what his followers should do after he was gone. The Buddha answered they should take responsibility for themselves ("be a lamp onto yourself"), guided by his teachings and the truth. The Buddha didn't want anyone to blindly adopt his way; he never asked anyone to accept his teaching until they had given it a thorough investigation. He wasn't looking to develop a following, but to open minds and hearts. He gave a method and guidelines, not answers.

We will always face decisions and situations that test our integrity and judgment, leaving us in some way, on our own, knowing death is our ultimate destination. Regardless of what system or method of navigation we do or don't use as we wind our way toward this ending, we should never discard our trusted guides of awareness, kindness, courage, and honesty.

Near the end of a 10-day course, S.N. Goenka tells the story of a mother who serves her son a scrumptious pudding filled with raisins, fruit, and other goodies. The boy likes the treat, but is suspicious of the "black stones" in the dish. "They're raisins," his mother tells him, "try them, they're delicious." But the boy refuses. And so it goes with the other sweet condiments in the dessert. He likes the pudding, but doesn't want to swallow all of it. The mother doesn't mind; she's content that he's basically happy. She also knows that as he grows up he will enjoy the rest. The moral: take what you can from what the Buddha has offered; don't worry about the parts you can't accept, perhaps someday they'll make sense to you.

After my first retreat ended, another first-timer said he initially liked this story, but then became offended because it was pejorative; it assumed that if you had any skepticism you were like an ignorant child. "So apply the *essence* of the story's message, its best part, to the story itself," I suggested. "Take what you feel is the wisdom in the parable and make use of that." By following this tact, we may still miss some kernels of truth—especially if we close ourselves off to words that don't jibe with our view—yet at least we'll be open to that wisdom for which we're ready, regardless of the packaging. In other words, we don't need to accept something whole hog to profit from it. In fact, if you believe that life is inherently dissatisfying, it's rare that we're going to be presented with the perfect parcel.

Yes, I am angling toward something. And that is that you don't need to accept everything that's been written in these pages to benefit from it. As I said in the introduction, my grand goal for this book is that it would inspire you to try a 10-day retreat (or, if you already have done one, to do them regularly). Almost everyone who takes one has a profound experience, even if they never do another retreat. And, as I hardly need to tell you, profound experiences are nothing to sneeze at. If the general gist of what you've read here makes sense, then, if I may be so bold, you owe it to yourself to at least try a course, even if you don't meditate regularly, or at all.

Even a long life is short. Ten days go by quickly. The moment is ripe, but may soon pass.

APPENDIX

TAKING A RETREAT

Just as a book about yoga can't truly replace taking yoga classes, this book can't truly be a substitute for spending ten days learning this method under the eye of an instructor. Indeed the best way to understand this method is by taking a ten-day course—which is designed to teach those new to this method. Although Mr. Goenka retired from presenting courses himself in the 1980s, the main instructions and talks at a course are given by him via audio and videotapes, with assistant teachers available at each course to give individualized guidance.

Mr. Goenka is a very skillful teacher. He's deft with tone and timing, and his words resonate with a much greater impact when heard than read. Mr. Goenka's power as a teacher reflects both his own depth of insight and his experience from instructing tens of thousands of students.

A ten-day course is the ideal setting for learning this technique. At a retreat you can be totally absorbed in meditating without your usual concerns. You don't have to worry about money, work, preparing meals, or doing chores. You'll be surrounded by other meditators putting out a strong effort, and of course it's helpful to have a teacher available to answer any questions you may have. This atmosphere makes it much easier to work with intent and intensity. On your own you'd be unlikely to meditate eleven hours a day for ten days. In fact, if you haven't done a retreat before, I'd strongly recommend against meditating for many hours a day on your own as you may experience unfamiliar or unsettling states of mind.* Yet, in the positively charged environment of a retreat, even people who've never meditated a whit before can manage sitting for the whole course and get great benefit from it.

Not surprisingly, this concentrated, consistent effort allows you to go deeper into the technique than if you practice on your own. So remember that any glimpses of peacefulness and insight you find from doing this on your own will be added to and multiplied many-fold on a retreat. In other words, you haven't truly given the method a fair chance until you do a course.

To take a 10-day course, contact one of the North American meditation centers listed on the following page. They will send you information that includes a schedule of available courses, what your daily schedule will be, and other details about rules and expectations. You can also find more information about this method and centers worldwide through the website www.dhamma.org

---

* Although it's unlikely meditating on your own, even a couple hours a day, would land you in unnerving psychological territory, if you do find yourself shaken, take a break and do something that grounds you, like talking to someone, going for a walk, or just focusing on your breath. No one ever got hurt from meditating, although if you have a mental disorder, I advise against doing this on your own.

ℚ

MAIN CENTERS IN NORTH AMERICA

• Vipassana Meditation Center
P.O. Box 24, Shelburne Falls, MA 01370
413-625-2160. Fax: 413-625-2170
info@dhara.dhamma.org

• California Vipassana Center
P.O. Box 1167, North Fork, CA 93643
559-877-4386. Fax 559- 877-4387
info@mahavana.dhamma.org

• Northwest Vipassana Center
P.O. Box 345, Ethel, WA 98542
360-978-5434. Fax: 360-978-5433
info@kunja.dhamma.org

• Southwest Vipassana Meditation Center
P.O. Box 190248, Dallas, TX 75219
214-521-5258. Fax: 214-522-5973
info@siri.dhamma.org

• Quebec Vipassana Meditation Center
P.O. Box 32083, Les Antriums, Montreal, QC H2l-4Y5
514-481-3504. Fax: 515-879-3437
info@suttama.dhamma.org

• Vipassana Meditation Center, BC
Box 529, Cambie, Vancouver, BC V5Z-4R3
604-730-9877. 604-641-2801
info@surabhi.dhamma.org

At this writing, there are also eleven satellite centers offering occasional or once a year 10-day courses in various spots throughout the U.S. Check the website www.dhamma.org or one of the main centers listed above for details.

Keep in mind this organization is run by volunteers, so responses to your inquiries may not be immediate.

SELECTED BIBLIOGRAPHY

Austin, James. *Zen and the Brain*. Cambridge: MIT Press, 1999.

Batchelor, Stephen. *Buddhism Without Beliefs*. New York: Riverhead Books, 1997.

Bercholz, Samuel and Kohn, Sherab Chödzin, editors. *Entering the Stream*. Boston: Shambhala Publications, 1993.

Bhikkhu Bodhi. *The Middle Length Discourses of the Buddha*. Boston: Wisdom Publications, 1995.

Briggs, John and Peat, David. *Seven Life Lessons of Chaos*. New York: HarperCollins, 1999.

Buddhist Publication Society. *Egolessness: Collected Essays*. Kandy, Sri Lanka: Buddhist Publication Society, 1984.

Capra, Fritjof. *The Tao of Physics*. New York: Bantam, 1975.

Dalai Lama and Cutler, Howard. *The Art of Happiness*. New York: Riverhead Books, 1998.

Darling, David. *The Zen of Physics*. New York: Harper Collins, 1996.

Das, Surya. *Awakening the Buddha Within*. New York: Broadway Books, 1997.

de Silva, Lily. Nibbana *As Living Experience*. Kandy, Sri Lanka: Buddhist Publication Society, 1996.

Dennett, Daniel. *Consciousness Explained*. Boston: Little Brown & Co., 1991.

Epstein, Mark. *Thoughts Without a Thinker*. New York: Basic Books, 1995.

Fields, Rick. *How the Swans Came to the Lake*. Boston: Shambhala Publications, 1992.

Fleischman, Paul. *Cultivating Inner Peace*. New York: Tarcher, 1997.

Fleischman, Paul. *Karma and Chaos*. Seattle: Vipassana Research Publications, 1999.

Flickstein, Matthew. *Journey to the Center*. Boston: Wisdom Publications, 1998.

Flickstein, Matthew. *Swallowing the River Ganges*. Boston: Wisdom Publications, 2001.

Glickman, Marshall. *The Mindful Money Guide.* New York: Ballantine Books. 1999.

Goenka, S.N. *The Discourse Summaries.* Seattle: Vipassana Research Publications, 1998.

Goenka, S.N. *Satipatthana Sutta Discourse.* Seattle: Vipassana Research, Publications, 1998.

Goldstein, Joseph and Kornfield, Jack. *Seeking the Heart of Wisdom.* Boston: Shambhala Publications, 1987.

Goleman, Daniel. *Emotional Intelligence.* New York: Bantam Books, 1995.

Goleman, Daniel. *The Meditative Mind.* New York: Tarcher, 1988.

Gunaratatana, Henepola. *Eight Mindful Steps to Happiness.* Boston: Wisdom Publications, 2001.

Gunaratatana, Henepola. *Mindfulness in Plain English.* Boston: Wisdom Publications, 1991.

Hagen, Steve. *Buddhism Plain and Simple.* Boston: Tuttle Publishing, 1997.

Hanh, Thich Nhat. *For a Future to be Possible.* Berkeley, CA: Parallax Press, 1998.

Hart, William. *The Art of Living.* San Francisco: Harper San Francisco, 1987.

Hayward, Jeremy. *Letters to Vanessa.* Boston: Shambhala Publications, 1997.

Hayward, Jeremy. *Shifting Worlds Changing Minds.* Boston: Shambhala Publications, 1987.

Johnson, Will. *The Posture of Meditation.* Boston: Shambhala Publications, 1996.

Kornfield, Jack. *After the Ecstacy, the Laundry.* New York: Bantam Books, 2001.

Kornfield, Jack. *Living Dharma.* Boston: Shambhala Publications, 1996.

Kornfield, Jack. *A Path With Heart.* New York: Bantam Books, 1993.

Krishnamurti, J. *Freedom From the Known.* New York: Harper & Row, 1969.

LeDoux, Joseph. *The Emotional Brain.* New York: Touchstone, 1996.

Levine, Stephen. *A Gradual Awakening.* New York: Anchor Books, 1979.

Macy, Joanna. *Mutual Causality in Buddhism and General Systems Theory.* Albany: State University of New York Press, 1991.

Nisker, Wes. *Buddha's Nature.* New York: Bantam Books, 1998.

Pinker, Steven. *How the Mind Works.* New York: W.W. Norton, 1997.

Rahula, Walpola. *What the Buddha Taught.* New York: Grove Weidenfeld, 1974.

Rapaport, Al, editor. *Buddhism in America.* Boston: Tuttle Publishing, 1998.

Revel, Jean-Francois and Ricard, Matthieu. *The Monk and the Philosopher.* New York: Schocken Books, 1999.

Smith, Huston. *The Religions of Man.* New York: Harper & Row, 1986.

Thanissaro Bhikkhu. *The Mind Like Fire Unbound.* Barre, MA: Dhamma Dana Publications, 1993.

Thomas, Lewis. *The Lives of a Cell.* New York: Bantam, 1974.

Varela, Francisco, Thompson, Evan, and Rosch, Eleanor. *The Embodied Mind.* Cambridge: MIT Press, 1996.

Vipassana Research Publications. *Mahasatipatthana Sutta.* Seattle: Vipassana Research Publications, 1996.

Walshe, Maurice. *The Long Discourses of the Buddha.* Boston: Wisdom Publications, 1995.

Welwood, John. *Toward a Psychology of Awakening.* Boston: Shambhala Publications, 2000.

Wilber, Ken. *No Boundary.* Boston: Shambhala Publications, 1985.

Wolf, Fred Alan. *Taking the Quantum Leap.* New York: Harper & Row, 1989.

Wright, Robert. *The Moral Animal.* New York: Vintage, 1994.

Wright, Robert. *Nonzero.* New York: Pantheon, 2000.

Zukav, Gary. *The Dancing Wu Li Masters.* New York: Bantam, 1980.

ACKNOWLEDGMENTS

I'd like to thank the following people:

Sarah Jane Freymann, my agent, who edited and helped shape the proposal, found a publisher (or two) for the book, and was always charming, even when I asked mundane questions.

Beth Umland, my sister-in-law, who is both family and one of my closest friends—although what she did for this book went beyond friendship and verged toward saintliness. When I first handed Beth my "final draft," I didn't realize how rickety it was. But like a combination architect, carpenter, and t'ai chi master, she helped shape it into something solid by knowing what needed detailing, what needed remodeling, and what called for outright demolition. That she was able to do all this with good humor while also managing a high-powered job and hectic family life (and no doubt also whipping through a few other books at the same time), is a testament to her intelligence and innate wisdom. As a mutual friend with Hindu leanings said of Beth, "She is an old soul."

Susan Gunther-Mohr for reading the karma chapter and giving valuable feedback.

Ben Gleason and Ed Walters, Tuttle editors, who gave many wise and thoughtful suggestions to make this book considerably more reader-friendly. And, Ashley Benning, for patiently answering my many questions about the copyedited manuscript and inputting my changes.

Jennifer Radalin, for adding clarity with her excellent copyediting and for weaning me from an inordinate fondness for quotation marks. And Linda Carey for her elegant text design.

Margaret Wimberger, my wife, for editing help and especially for tolerating my many late and weekend hours at the computer.

Likewise, I thank and apologize to Soph and Lena Bean for putting up with lost dad time.

INDEX

A

Abhidhamma, 15
acceptance, 58–60, 63–65,
     77–78; and ego,
     191; and karma,
     139; and pain,
     167–68
addiction, 159, 170–73;
     treating, 173–77.
     See also pleasure
After the Ecstasy, the
     Laundry
     (Kornfield), 205
altruism, 122–23
ānāpāna, 83–85, 87–91
Aristotle, 159
Armstrong, Karen, 191
Art of Living, The, 8
atoms, qualities of, 183–84
attachment, 61–62
attitude, in meditation,
     76–78
Awakening of the West: The
     Encounter of
     Buddhism and
     Western Culture
     (Batchelor), 195
awareness, 31–32, 39,
     67–68; and ego,
     191; and equanim-
     ity, 69–70, 76; and
     karma, 139; and
     pleasure, 162; of

sensations, xii, 35,
     43–46, 104–5,
     113–15. *See also*
     mindfulness

B

Batchelor, Stephen, 16, 37,
     38, 145, 195
Baumeister, Roy F., 190
Being Nobody, Going
     Nowhere (Khema),
     27
bhanga (dissolution), 97
Bhikkhu Bodhi, 114
body: and equanimity,
     70–71; meditation
     posture, 81–83;
     mind and emotions,
     xii, 47–52, 134–36;
     and pleasure/pain,
     163–66, 169–70;
     scan, in meditation,
     92–100; and uncon-
     scious, 52–54
brain, processing of,
     185–86, 187
breath: ānāpāna, 83–85,
     87–91; focusing on,
     41, 113–14
Brief History of Everything,
     A (Wilber), 119
Buddha, 2–3; on change,
     14; on doubt/effort,